Hypertension
A Policy Perspective

HYPERTENSION
A Policy Perspective

Milton C. Weinstein
William B. Stason

with contributions by
David Blumenthal
Barbara J. McNeil
Albert L. Nichols
Donald S. Shepard

Harvard University Press
Cambridge, Massachusetts
London, England
1976

Library of Congress Cataloging in Publication Data

Weinstein, Milton C
    Hypertension : a policy perspective.
    Bibliography: p.
    Includes index.
    1.   Hypertension—Economic aspects—United States.
2.   Hypertension—Prevention—Cost effectiveness.
3.   Hypertension—United States—Prevention.   I.   Stason,
William B., joint author.   II.   Title.   [DNLM:
1.   Hypertension.   WG340 W424h]
RA645.H9W43   362.1′9′613200973   76-25881
ISBN 0-674-43900-7

To Rhonda and Susan

Foreword

Until recently, the only important professional interface involving the medical profession and the lay public was that between the doctor and the patient. That relationship, of course, remains and will always be of crucial importance. However, a combination of factors has now served to focus attention on a second area of critical interaction—that between medicine and society. The allocation of health resources, legal and ethical aspects of medical care and of experimentation in human subjects, the role of technology in medical care, problems of access to medical care, the assessment of quality of care—these and many more issues increasingly occupy the attention not only of physicians but of other professionals, the press, decision makers, and the public at large. Several reasons may be cited: the concern of the consumer movement with issues of medical practice; a recognition that we do not have adequate resources to provide everything in medical care of which we are capable; an awareness of inequities in the allocation of resources; a greater appreciation of both the natural history of disease and the effectiveness and limitations of intervention; and a growing recognition that many skills in addition to medical ones can have extremely important effects on health.

Several efforts are under way to bring together people whose thoughtful deliberations can contribute to consideration and resolution of these complex issues. One approach recently undertaken at Harvard was the establishment of the Center for the Analysis of Health Practices. Based in the School of Public Health, this center attracts professionals from throughout the university, including physicians, policy analysts, economists, lawyers, ethicists, statisticians, experts in management, and many others. Small groups have been constituted to deal with a variety of health problems. Typically, such groups assess the state of the art, then pose the principal questions that confront society, and, finally, use existing data to lay out the options for immediate or future action. Throughout the process, efforts are made to establish and maintain close contacts with interested groups outside the University, particularly those making public policy decisions.

This book is one of the first products of the center. It represents the fruits of a collaboration between Dr. Weinstein, a policy analyst from the School of Public Health and the Kennedy School of Government, and Dr. Stason, a cardiologist from the School of Public Health and the Medical School. The history of their interaction is instructive. In advance of their meeting, neither had more than a passing acquaintance with the discipline of the other. Each discovered that he needed a prolonged period of intensive interaction to achieve an understanding of the other's profession, including its language and approach. Dr. Weinstein early appreciated that medical decisions are frequently made by physicians who do not have access to the combined experience of large numbers of other physicians, to comprehensive analysis of that experience, and to careful consideration of the options for reasonable action suggested by that experience. Consequently, the physician often is not in a position to suggest the optimal strategy for the patient in question. Moreover, Dr. Weinstein soon discovered many ways in which the interests of the individual patient conflict with the interests of society, a dilemma long appreciated by the physician caring for that patient and, of course, resolved by the physician in favor of the patient. Dr. Stason, in turn, quickly saw the pitfalls inherent in even the most sophisticated policy analysis when undertaken without adequate medical data and without full appreciation of the nuances of the patient/doctor interaction. During the course of their work, both came to realize what the other's discipline and perspective could offer, and that a collaborative enterprise might be much more meaningful than the sum of the individual contributions.

This volume is considered by my policy-analyst colleagues as representing very distinguished policy research. As a physician, I am unable to contribute to this evaluation. However, it is apparent to me that this volume could have profound effects. The illness with which it deals is one of the most common afflicting Americans. Hypertension can now be effectively treated, and there is overwhelming evidence that such treatment can prevent serious complications in a sizeable fraction of those afflicted.

For the physician and the individual with hypertension confronted with important decisions in clinical management, this book offers background that will help replace dogma with a reasoned analysis of existing information. Clearly, it is not intended to replace the judgment of the physician in planning a treatment program for the patient. However, it will arm physician and patient with those facts that are known and provide help in interpreting and applying them to specific problems.

For public and policy makers the book provides information required for decisions concerning allocation of resources for screening programs, treatment programs, and further research.

For students of the disease it lays out the gaps in our knowledge that require further research and analysis. For example, the authors point to the need for improved methods of data collection. They focus also on the inadequacies of our understanding of human behavior. In hypertension as in many other health problems, we are increasingly aware that if patients would act in their own self interest, they could do much to improve health. The book indicates the perils of strategies that take for granted compliance with recommendations for treatment. In addition, it points to the urgent need for designing better antihypertensive drugs.

And finally, for the medical profession and for the many other professionals and students now increasingly interested in health problems, this work will serve as a paradigm for the systematic analysis of other important health practices. The absence of such analyses has been costly in money, human suffering, and lives. Consider, for example, the number of medical practices that have been in vogue for long periods, only to be abandoned when shown to be useless. We are now embarked on a national program designed to deal with the problem of hypertension. This program, in contrast to some others, has been carefully conceived and analyzed. Several professionals involved in the national effort have acknowledged that the perspectives provided in this volume could significantly affect their future decisions. If the approach presented by Drs. Weinstein and Stason is adopted as a model for other national or local programs designed to deal with medical problems, additional great benefits could ensue.

Howard H. Hiatt, M.D.
Dean
Harvard School of Public Health

Preface

From the time the Center for the Analysis of Health Practices (CAHP) was organized in 1973, one of its primary objectives was to foster interdisciplinary policy studies of important problems in health and medicine. As two of CAHP's first members, we embodied this interdisciplinary ideal: a quantitatively oriented policy analyst with no medical training and a cardiologist with no experience in quantitative policy analysis. What we had in common at that time, though, was the desire to join forces to address an important medical problem from our combined perspectives, with the hope of generating insights that could not have been generated by either one of us alone. We chose hypertension because it is a major public health problem for which effective treatment is available but not optimally applied, because it already attracts considerable health care resources and has the potential for attracting a great deal more, because governments and health institutions at all levels are devoting increased attention to it, and because the data on its prevalence and associated risks are relatively good compared to many other medical conditions.

Our purposes in setting out on the study were threefold: to demonstrate the usefulness of systematic policy analysis in addressing the issues of resource allocation that surround a complex, uncertainty-laden medical detection and treatment problem; to stimulate others to attempt similar analyses of other medical problems so that a basis for allocating resources among diseases can be established; and to awaken physicians, and others involved in health care, to the reality of limited resources and to offer a rational approach to decision making that recognizes this reality.

Preparation of this volume was assisted by a grant from The Robert Wood Johnson Foundation, Princeton, New Jersey. The opinions, conclusions, and proposals in the text are those of the authors and do not necessarily represent the views of The Robert Wood Johnson Foundation.

On a different level, this study provided the opportunity to test the viability of interdisciplinary research. This was a saga unto itself. Initially, communication between us was limited by our lack of understanding of each other's analytical viewpoint. With perseverence, however, we gradually taught each other enough about our respective disciplines to function as a team. Each chapter, and even each page, represents a joint effort and could not have been written by either one of us alone, at least not until the process of mutual immersion in each other's professional worlds had run its course.

An important function of a project such as this in a university setting is to provide a link between the research activities of faculty and the education of students. We were fortunate to involve several students in this study as part of their graduate training in public policy analysis at the Kennedy School of Government. Of these, three produced papers that led to parts of this book. David Blumenthal, while also a fourth year medical student, prepared an analysis of the side effects of thiazide diuretics and reserpine as a term exercise in his training in policy analysis. We extended this analysis to include methyldopa and adapted it to the analytical framework of the book to create chapter 3. A. L. Nichols, also a student at the Kennedy School, formulated the resource allocation model upon which chapter 6 rests. Donald Shepard, as part of his doctoral dissertation in public policy, conceptualized the use of financial incentives to affect patient behavior. His contribution is incorporated in chapter 4. Two other Kennedy School students made important contributions to our research effort that were not directly included in the book but served as important resource documents. Kathryn Bernick spent a summer analyzing the characteristics and performance of hypertension screening programs around the country, and Albert Mulley evaluated the role of professional education in promoting the control of hypertension.

Our other major collaborator was a radiologist who has pioneered the use of quantitative analysis in medical decision making. Barbara McNeil provided the technical basis for the analysis of renovascular disease in chapter 7 and helped us develop it into its final form.

Throughout our effort, no person was more helpful or more supportive than Howard Hiatt, Dean of the Harvard School of Public Health. His encouragement and his assistance in circumventing obstacles were indispensible.

Soon after Howard Frazier became the director of CAHP in September 1975, he pushed the book forward as one of the highest priorities of the center, urged us on toward timely publication, offered many helpful suggestions to improve the manuscript, and freed the required secretarial time. With his support, our confidence level rose and publication quickly became a reality.

We are grateful to many other people who have helped to improve the content of the book by giving of their time in helpful discussions and by providing us with critical comments. Early on, Peter Braun helped us to settle on hypertension as the target of our efforts and provided insightful suggestions from the perspective of the practicing clinician. Robert Levy and his staff at the National Heart and Lung Institute took time out from their busy schedules to discuss our studies with us and to give us their written comments on one of the drafts. We were indeed fortunate to benefit from their unique perspectives. Discussions with Shan Cretin and Donald Berwick, who were just beginning a parallel policy study relating to serum cholesterol screening for children, were helpful in developing the analytic models for our analysis. Arthur Dempster and Richard Zeckhauser gave us thoughtful comments that helped us to adapt the text to the needs of our diverse readers.

The typing of the manuscript was a true happening. Sue Kaufman and Laurie Pearlman interspersed hours of flawless typing with moments of real delight for all of us. We shall never forget the first performance of the medley of tunes they composed in our honor, including "The Sphygmomanometer with the Fringe on Top" and also the following, sung to the tune of "Oklahoma," which we cannot refrain from sharing with our readers, and which we quote with the permission of the composers:

> Hy . . . pertension,
> When the blood comes rushin' down the veins [sic],
> It's not enough to screen,
> You must intervene,
> 'Cause you know adherence is a pain!
>
> Cost . . . effective-
> ness is what this book is all about,
> If we screen them all and treat them all,
> We are throwing public monies out.

We know intervention is best,
Even discounted it passes the test!
So when we say "quality-adjusted life years" we're only
    saying
You're doin' fine while you're livin'
If your adherence
Is okay.

Such talent has to be heard to be fully appreciated.

One of the most awe-inspiring tasks imaginable is the compilation and verification of a bibliography; Eleanor Druckman performed this job admirably. Other staff members at the Center for the Analysis of Health Practices to whom we owe thanks include Carol Weisberg and Maureen Rush, who provided cheerful and expert typing assistance; Jody Mighill, who orchestrated the overall production process; and Kathleen Ittner, who saw to it that our every administrative need was met. In addition, we deeply appreciate the generosity of our colleagues at the center who agreed to postpone the production of their own materials so that ours could be expedited.

Finally, we are grateful to The Robert Wood Johnson Foundation and the Commonwealth Fund for their financial support of our work at the Center for the Analysis of Health Practices.

Boston   Milton C. Weinstein, Ph.D.
May 1976   William B. Stason, M.D., S.M.

Contents

Tables

Figures

Hypertension
A Policy Perspective

1. Introduction

One of America's foremost health problems is hypertension, or high blood pressure, a malady that affects between ten and thirty percent of the adult population of the United States. It is the most important single risk factor for that class of disease—cardiovascular disease—that kills and cripples more people than any other. Effective treatment is available but infrequently applied. Furthermore it is estimated that treatment, if provided for all hypertensives, would be expensive: nearly five billion dollars a year or four percent of total current health expenditures in the United States. For these reasons, public policy toward the treatment of hypertension is an important concern.

A half century ago, this policy analysis would not have been written. In the first place, hypertension was at that time ill-defined, of uncertain significance, and not amenable to interventions; moreover, it was overwhelmed in importance by the most pressing health problem of the day, infectious disease. Second, the costs of health care constituted a relatively smaller part of the national economy and, because they were defrayed predominantly from private sources, commanded less public attention. Third, the art and science of public policy analysis did not exist, not only because the requisite mathematical and economic tools had not been developed, but also because there had not yet been felt a critical need for a systematic approach to public decision making and resource allocation. As we enter the last quarter of the twentieth century, all three of these conditions have changed dramatically.

During the last twenty to thirty years a variety of quantitative techniques have been developed to analyze decision problems. Falling under the rubric of operations research, management science, or, more broadly, systems analysis, these methods have been applied successfully in the areas of national defense and private business. More recently, they have been joined with those

1

of applied economics and political science to address a wide range of public policy problems that had previously escaped systematic decision-oriented analysis. This study represents an attempt to combine this analytical perspective with that of clinical medicine in addressing a major categorical health problem. As such it may serve as a model for similar evaluations of other health problems.

Throughout, the attempt is made to be sensitive to the range of values and criteria that enter into health policy decision making. The perspective taken is that of society, defined here as the aggregate of individuals who compose the United States population. Since most members of society use the health care system and also help to pay for it, they have an interest in both the benefits it provides and the costs it entails.

Criteria to be considered in selecting a policy include efficiency, equity, and political feasibility. Efficiency refers to the policy imperative that, under conditions of limited resources, benefits should be achieved at the least possible resource cost. Equivalently, available resources should be allocated among alternative uses to achieve the maximum benefit possible. These considerations apply to allocations within a categorical problem such as hypertension, to allocations among competing health programs, and to allocations between health programs and other uses of resources. The definition of benefits derived from health programs is, obviously, a related issue, and variations in individual preferences for health and health care need to be taken into account. A second criterion is that of equity. The distribution of the benefits and costs of health care among the members of society is to be valued as well as the aggregate of benefits and costs. Unlike efficiency, however, equity carries no clear definition of what is good or bad. The best one can do is to describe the distributional implications of alternative policies, since it would be impossible to rank these distributions unambiguously on a scale of equity. This analysis does consider equity in several contexts, including that between those whose concern for their health causes them to seek health care and undertake preventive actions on their own, and those who do not. A third criterion, like it or not, is political feasibility. Any policy must be evaluated in the light of practical considerations embodied in the legislative and administrative processes of government and health care institutions. These considerations are alluded to wherever possible in the course of the analysis and underlie the resulting recommendations.

For many reasons, the decisions made by individuals and organizations in the health care sector are not always in accord with the social criteria of efficiency and equity. Divergence occurs in part because patients expect and demand high quality medical care when they need it but pay the price for their collective behavior only indirectly through insurance premiums and taxes. It also stems in part from the fact that the professional objectives and personal needs of providers, and the institutional goals of the organizations in which they practice, are often in conflict with the long-term health and financial interests of society. Agents of society are needed to intervene to correct these divergences: government may act through health insurance reimbursement packages, quality assurance criteria, and state and local service programs, while community and professional groups operate through service, education, and peer review programs. Throughout this analysis, when objectives held by individual decision makers tend to lead to practices that are at odds with the best interests of society, possible reasons will be discussed. From these will follow implications for the implementation of recommended strategies for the management of hypertension.

Hypertension, the Medical Problem

Hypertension is no more, and no less, than high arterial blood pressure. Despite the associations conjured up by the name, it does not imply any psychological syndrome; frequently, in fact, there are no outward manifestations, either physical or emotional. Furthermore, hypertension is not a disease but simply a quantitative deviation of blood pressure relative to the norm in a population. Some people have higher blood pressure than others, and the higher one's blood pressure the greater the risk of subsequent cardiovascular disease.

On a physiological level, blood pressure depends upon the resistance to the flow of blood through the arteries and upon cardiac output. It varies during each contraction of the heart from a maximum when the heart is most contracted (systole) to a minimum when it is most relaxed (diastole).[1] In the United States adult population, systolic pressures of 120 millimeters of mercury (mm Hg) and diastolic pressures of 80 mm Hg are average. By convention, but without any implication of a discrete physiological basis for the cutoff point, blood pressures above 160/95 (that is, over 160 mm Hg systolic and/or over 95 mm Hg diastolic) are usually designated as hypertensive [National High Blood Pressure Education Program, 1973b].

Blood pressure is a rather elusive quantity, varying widely from time to time within the course of the day and from day to day. It is usually lowest in the morning or when one is relaxed, and highest late in the afternoon or during times of stress. These vicissitudes pose problems for accurate measurement and for diagnosis.

The first measurement of blood pressure in man was made using an instrument developed by Hérisson in 1834. This consisted of "a metal hemisphere sealed on its plane surface with a flexible membrane and carrying a graduated capillary tube at its summit. The apparatus was filled with mercury to part way up the capillary. When placed over the radial artery, the pulsations were transmitted to the capillary tube where they could be measured" [Pickering, 1955]. Today, arterial pressures in humans can be measured most accurately by inserting a needle or catheter into an artery and attaching it to a manometer. Such a procedure is invasive and expensive, however, and is impractical for routine clinical use. Instead, indirect measurement by a procedure developed by Riva-Rocci in 1896 is usually employed, in which "a soft rubber cuff in a more rigid cloth case is applied to the upper arm and inflated to a pressure which obliterates the pulse; the pressure is allowed to fall until the pulse returns. The pressure is measured by a mercury manometer" [Pickering, 1968]. This apparatus, known as a sphygmomanometer, has become as intrinsic a part of the physician's tool kit as the stethoscope. More recently, automated sphygmomanometers, devices to measure blood pressure by passing ultrasonic waves through the arm, and coin-operated machines with digital readout have been developed and are becoming available to the public.

---

1. Mean arterial pressure, which is a weighted average of blood pressure throughout the cardiac cycle, is often a useful concept, but is difficult to measure directly. Mean pressures usually approximate the weighted average: $(2/3 \times \text{diastolic pressure}) + (1/3 \times \text{systolic pressure})$.

CAUSES

Despite intensive research, the causes of hypertension remain poorly understood. More than 95 percent of hypertensive Americans have what is labeled "essential hypertension," meaning simply that the elevation in blood pressure cannot be traced to any known cause. Familial aggregation studies suggest that both genetic and environmental factors play roles in the etiology of essential hypertension [Zinner et al., 1975; Feinleib et al., 1975]. The possible implication of salt intake has been raised by a variety of cross-cultural studies that show lower levels of blood pressure in populations with low salt consumption [Page, Damon, and Moellering, 1974; Shaper, 1972], but relationships between blood pressure and salt intake within populations have been equivocal [Knudson, Iwai, and Dahl, 1973; Miall and Oldham, 1958]. In addition, psychological stress has been cited as a possible contributing cause of hypertension [Gutmann and Benson, 1971; Henry and Cassel, 1969].

In a minority of patients with hypertension, a specific underlying condition, such as a malfunctioning kidney or tumor of the adrenal gland, can be identified. In such cases of "secondary hypertension," specific and frequently curative treatments are often possible, though at the cost of sophisticated diagnostic detective work and expensive surgical procedures.

The primary focus in this analysis is on essential hypertension, though issues involved in the diagnosis and treatment of secondary hypertension are discussed in chapter 7.

RISKS

Clinical consequences of high blood pressure manifest themselves primarily in the brain, the heart, and the kidneys. In the brain, strokes result either from the rupture of blood vessels (hemorrhagic strokes) or their occlusion by atheromatous material (thrombotic strokes). In the heart, exertional chest pain (angina pectoris) and heart attack (myocardial infarction) are manifestations of the coronary artery disease that develops at an accelerated rate in hypertensive individuals. At the same time, the strain imposed on the heart by elevated blood pressure, with or without coronary artery disease, may lead to congestive heart failure. Kidney failure due to arteriosclerosis of renal blood vessels is another possible consequence. All of these conditions are accompanied by a significant risk of death and considerable morbidity.

Reliable quantitative data on the risks of death and disease associated with the level of blood pressure were first made available in 1959 by the Build and Blood Pressure Study of the Society of Actuaries [1959–1960]. This landmark study, based on information from 3.9 million policyholders between 1935 and 1954, is still used by the insurance industry for underwriting purposes [Lew, 1973; National Heart and Lung Institute, 1974]. The interest of the insurance industry in the effects of high blood pressure is itself an indication of the magnitude of the problem. More recently data from long-term studies of defined communities such as the Framingham Heart Study [Dawber, Meadors, and Moore, 1951] and the Tecumseh Study [Epstein, Ostrander, and Johnson, 1965] have provided additional valuable insights into the risks of stroke, heart attack, and other events in relation to blood pressure.

Hypertension is a particularly troublesome risk factor for cardiovascular disease because of its insidious nature: it is usually without symptoms during most of its clinical course. Thus, unless a person has his blood pressure measured, he will be unaware of the potential risks he faces. Exceptions exist, as in the case of so-called "malignant" or "accelerated" hypertension, in which the blood pressure is acutely and dangerously elevated, but such cases are relatively rare. Headaches, which were once thought to be a characteristic symptom, are now generally believed to result from anxiety associated with the awareness of hypertension or from unrelated nonspecific causes [Pickering, 1968].

TREATMENT

At the present time, the objective of treatment for essential hypertension is to lower arterial blood pressure. Better understanding of the causes of hypertension is required before specific preventive or curative measures can be developed. Until that time, antihypertensive drugs will remain the mainstay of therapy. Adjunctive efforts to limit salt intake, to encourage an obese patient to lose weight, and to reduce stress by such means as the "relaxation response" [Benson et al., 1974; Patel and North, 1975] may facilitate management, and reduction in other risk factors for cardiovascular disease, such as high serum cholesterol and cigarette smoking, may be of additional benefit.

In the early 1950s, hexamethonium and related drugs were first used in the treatment of malignant hypertension. A few years later, a class of drugs known as diuretics was developed and applied to hypertension, and then during the 1960s an ever increasing array of drugs based on a variety of pharmacological principles became available. Drugs in common use today are the diuretics (chiefly thiazide derivatives), the rauwolfia alkaloids (reserpine), the vasodilators (hydralazine), alpha-methyldopa, adrenergic blocking agents (guanethidine), and the beta-blockers (propranolol). These aim to decrease blood pressure by reducing vascular resistance, by lowering cardiac output, or both. To maintain blood pressure at a lower level, drug use almost always must be continued for the rest of one's life.

The value of lowering blood pressures in patients with malignant hypertension was clearly demonstrated in the late 1950s [Dustan et al., 1958; Harrington, Kincaid-Smith, and McMichael, 1959; Sokolow and Perloff, 1960; Bjork et al., 1961; Mohler and Freis, 1960]. Several years passed, however, before any significant evidence was obtained that treatment of milder hypertension is effective in reducing the risks that high blood pressure creates. In 1964, Hamilton showed that blood pressure reduction from diastolic levels averaging 110 mm Hg and higher was beneficial in reducing risk in both men and women [Hamilton, 1966]. More recently, the Veterans Administration Cooperative Study found that blood pressure reduction was effective in men, at least for those with initial diastolic pressures of 105 mm Hg or higher [1967, 1970]. While some doubt still remains as to the generalizability of these findings, this study has been largely responsible for bringing hypertension into the national spotlight as a public health problem to be reckoned with.

Unfortunately, antihypertensive treatment is not a free ride. Side effects of medications range from minor and transient problems such as lethargy, diarrhea, skin rash, and nausea to severe and disabling problems such as impotence, depression, and possibly cancer. Moreover, the drugs and associated medical supervision cost from $100 to $500 per patient per year, equivalent to many thousands of dollars over a lifetime. The pros and cons of treatment must be weighed carefully by the physician and by the policy maker alike in deciding what initiatives are justified.

Hypertension, the Public Health Problem

In 1964 it was estimated that about 17 percent of the American adult population had blood pressures above 160/95 mm Hg [National Center for Health Statistics, 1964a]. Extrapolated to 1976, this means that 24 million persons—11 million men and 13 million women—are hypertensive. An additional 23 million have blood pressures above 140/90 but below 160/95. Thus nearly one of three American adults is either hypertensive or on the threshold of becoming hypertensive. On the basis of prevalence alone, hypertension is unrivaled among major health problems.

The number of deaths and illnesses attributable to hypertension is also impressive. While hypertension was listed as the primary cause of over 65,000 deaths in 1966, this figure grossly underestimates its total impact on mortality. A major fraction of the more than 1 million annual deaths due to diseases of the circulatory system also can be attributed to hypertension, as can a major fraction of the more than 1.5 million nonfatal strokes and heart attacks per year. Because half of the hypertensives in the United States are under the age of 54, and more than 20 percent are under the age of 44, the implications of untreated hypertension for life expectancy are striking. This is particularly true for black Americans, a group for whom access to quality medical care has historically been limited, and who compose 18 percent of hypertensives, compared to only 9 percent of the total population.

For all of these reasons, hypertension is a public health problem of the first magnitude. Despite this, only about half of American hypertensives are even aware they have high blood pressure, only about one-fourth are under treatment, and only about one-eighth are receiving adequate blood pressure-lowering therapy. This evident failure of patients, health care providers, and the medical care system to accomplish effective treatment of 21 million of the 24 million hypertensives raises major public policy questions. On one hand, it can be argued that a major national effort should be undertaken to see to it that treatment is provided to as many of the untreated 21 million hypertensives as possible. On the other hand, treatment is costly (an estimated 4.8 billion dollars per year for 24 million hypertensives), is accompanied by side effects, and is of uncertain efficacy in the 70 to 80 percent of such individuals who have mild hypertension. Furthermore, considerable expenditures beyond pure treatment costs may be required to alter the health care system sufficiently to slow the attrition process.

WHAT IS BEING DONE ABOUT HYPERTENSION

Activities relating to hypertension in the United States can be classified into three broad areas: research, clinical practice, and public policy. Research into the causes and treatment of hypertension has been a primary thrust of academic medicine and the National Institutes of Health for several decades. Better definition of its pathophysiology and the development of a multitude of antihypertensive medications have been the results. Clinical practice has, in turn, been influenced by evolving knowledge. Diagnostic work-ups for rare causes of secondary hypertension have become commonplace. Physicians now are more aware of the importance of hypertension and the benefits of its treatment. There are still, however, many physicians who do not measure blood pressure routinely, and many more who do not treat hypertension when found. Likewise there are many patients who do not take medications when prescribed.

On the level of public policy, in July 1972 Secretary of Health, Education, and Welfare, Elliot Richardson, launched the National High Blood Pressure Education Program (NHBPEP), "a nationwide program of professional and public information designed to reduce the morbidity and mortality resulting from this disease in the United States" [National High Blood Pressure Education Program, 1973a]. Richardson placed responsibility for this program in the National Institutes of Health (NIH), particularly the National Heart and Lung Institute (NHLI). This choice was significant in that the focus and predisposition of the NHLI had previously been predominantly on biomedical research. At this time, however, it was given responsibility for federal action in the area of hypertension control. To facilitate the development and implementation of policy by the NHBPEP, two groups were created: the Hypertension Information and Education Advisory Committee, consisting of medical authorities from around the country, and the Interagency Working Group, consisting of representatives of relevant federal agencies. In September 1973 these groups produced the High Blood Pressure Education Plan based on the recommendations of four task forces. This consisted of simplified guidelines for clinical management of hypertension and for professional and community education, as well as a projection of the resource requirements of a nationwide campaign to control hypertension. As of 1976, the NHBPEP is in the process of implementing some of these recommendations. A public education program, operating on a very small budget, aims to educate the public about hypertension through media campaigns and to stimulate local and private educational efforts by providing teaching materials; a professional education program, involving a task group of medical educators, has devised criteria for the curricula of hypertension training programs and standards for evaluation [National High Blood Pressure Education Program, 1975]; and a community consultation service is available to state and local agencies seeking guidance in setting up their own hypertension control programs [Stokes and Ward, 1974]. These efforts are supplemented by controlled clinical trials such as the multicenter Hypertension Detection and Follow-up Program, which is attempting to resolve unanswered questions of treatment efficacy in a community setting. As of 1976, the federal government has not, however, become directly involved in programs to detect, treat, and manage hypertension. Such public programs as have existed have been initiated at the state and local levels and by private organizations such as the American Heart Association. Most of these have been on a small scale and short-term.

Hypertension, the Policy Problem

There are many reasons why hypertension has become a major area of public health policy concern in the United States and why the time is ripe for a systematic appraisal. First, as noted previously, the evidence is now clear that high blood pressure is the cause of a staggering amount of death and disability in the United States. Second, treatment has been shown to be beneficial for many patients; even skeptics are now convinced that hypertension is one of the few chronic conditions for which this is unequivocally so. Third, the increasing emphasis on cost control, stimulated by spiraling health care costs, has led to an increased commitment on the part of the government to foster careful evaluation of existing as well as new health programs. Accelerated efforts to control hypertension present both the possibility of major new benefits to the health of the American population and also the danger of expensive programs that further accelerate medical care inflation. Current interest in prepaid group practices, including health maintenance organizations, as well as the prospect of national health insurance, provide opportunities and incentives to examine the desirability of new health initiatives that compete for resources with other health services.

The ultimate determination of policy is complicated by the fact that no single decision maker or decision-making entity is in a position to enforce its implementation. Outcomes will be determined by the interaction of a number of decisions at the federal, state, and local levels of government, by fiscal intermediaries, by pharmacists and the pharmaceutical industry, and by the many people who make up the health care delivery system, including members of peer review organizations, clinic directors, hospital administrators, health maintenance organization administrators, physicians in private practice, and consumers. Each has unique interests and incentives that may lead to health practices different from those that society as a whole would choose. For example, patients with health insurance may overutilize medical services because the financial disincentives are minimal. Providers who are reimbursed on a fee-for-service basis rarely consider cost in their decision making, especially for patients who are insured. Moreover, because providers tend to derive more satisfaction from treating acute or symptomatic problems than from managing chronic or asymptomatic conditions, the former tend to be relatively overemphasized. Prepaid group practices such as health maintenance organizations, on the other hand, have ample incentives to control cost, but this may lead to underutilization, particularly when the patient has no symptoms demanding attention.

From the policy perspective, the focus of this analysis is on the resource allocation decisions that are or may be faced by these decision makers, albeit from different viewpoints. Among the questions are:

- Should major new resources be devoted to the treatment of hypertension?
- How should priorities for the use of treatment resources be set?
- How should the problem of drug side effects influence treatment and policy decisions?
- Considering that many patients do not adhere to medical

regimens, is treatment of hypertension nevertheless a wise use of resources?

• What kinds of public, provider, or patient educational programs should be implemented?

• Should hypertension screening programs be implemented? Under what conditions? For what target populations?

• How should resources be divided among screening, treatment, and follow-up interventions?

• How much effort should be spent in diagnosing the known curable forms of hypertension?

• What incentives can be provided to the patient, the provider, or other decision makers to encourage them to act in the public interest?

• When should action be taken on the basis of incomplete information, and when should the results of further research be awaited? What areas for research should have highest priority?

The Analytic Approach

The rationale for performing this analysis is that, since decisions must and will be made one way or another, they should be made in a systematic manner rather than on an ad hoc basis. It is hoped that the analytic framework presented will be useful to a wide range of decision makers. The fundamental approach taken is to subdivide the complex problem of hypertension management into its salient component parts, each of which is addressed individually. These parts are then combined and organized into a framework useful for decision making.

Structuring includes the specification of objectives (for example, reduced mortality, reduced costs), the definition of policy alternatives, and the combination of these into a model by which to measure the performance of alternative strategies. As noted previously, the objectives are taken to be aggregate health benefits and net costs to the United States society at large. The alternatives are primarily those faced by the various federal, state, and local governmental agencies and by community groups and professional organizations which act on behalf of the interests of the public or particular segments of the population. They also include actions available to fiscal intermediaries, providers, and patients.

Formulation of the model is based on the best data available. The medical literature is used to the maximal extent possible.

Where gaps in information exist, subjective estimates are used to supplement it. Though imperfect, the knowledge upon which the model is based does provide a rational basis for decision making.

Given these considerations, our conclusions clearly cannot be definitive. Though we believe that our assumptions are realistic, we recognize that different assumptions may lead to different conclusions. It is hoped that those who differ with the underlying assumptions or quantitative estimates will substitute their own estimates to derive their own conclusions. To assist in that regard, *sensitivity analysis* is performed in areas where the data are particularly soft, to determine which predicted outcomes are most sensitive to variations in parameters of the model and, therefore, which conclusions are most tenuous. Prime targets for research can thereby be identified.

Throughout, problems of implementation are considered by identifying the variety of perspectives of the decision makers involved and by probing the political implications of program strategies and the organizational and bureaucratic obstacles to change. New institutional structures just now being formulated, including national health insurance, quality assurance, and pre-paid practice, may facilitate implementation of socially optimal health practices.

This decision-oriented analysis of hypertension focuses on the problems of resource allocation. The major objective is to determine which allocation of available resources among and within intervention categories will result in the greatest health benefit, as measured by reductions in mortality and morbidity.

There are two general principles guiding efficient resource allocation. The first is that available health care resources be allocated among alternative uses to achieve the maximum total health benefit. This implies that priorities should be based on the health benefits produced per dollar spent and applies both to allocation within a categorical health problem such as hypertension and to tradeoffs between hypertension and other areas of health care. *Cost-effectiveness analysis* is a method used to apply this principle [Acton, 1973]. The second principle applies when resources need to be allocated between health and nonhealth programs. In this case, an allocation decision involves the valuation of health benefits relative to nonhealth benefits. For example, a decision to increase the national health budget to control

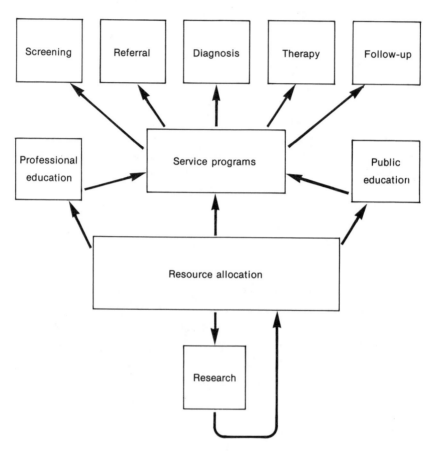

Figure 1.1: Broad areas of resource allocation for hypertension control.

hypertension would reflect the value judgment that it is worth more to spend the additional money on hypertension to achieve the resulting prolongation of life and improvement in its quality than to use it to produce other goods or services that people value. *Cost-benefit analysis* attempts to make these tradeoffs explicit [Weisbrod, 1961; Klarman, 1965; Acton, 1973].

This analysis expands upon these methodologies, primarily cost-effectiveness, by taking into account the uncertainty about both the effects and costs of alternative actions and by including valued outcomes such as quality of life that are usually ignored or given only passing reference in such analyses. It draws heavily from the techniques of *decision analysis* [Raiffa, 1968; Howard, 1968] to supplement the cost-effectiveness framework for resource allocation. Moreover, unlike much cost-effectiveness and

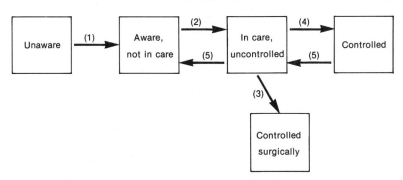

Figure 1.2: State-transition model for the analysis of hypertension policy. Interventions contributing to flows between states are designated as follows: (1) screening; (2) referral; (3) diagnosis; (4) therapy; (5) follow-up.

cost-benefit analysis, the intent is to be flexible in the formulation of assumptions and therefore in the statement of conclusions.

General areas that compete for resources in hypertension include service programs, educational programs, and research. Within service programs, major activities are screening, referral, diagnosis, therapy, and follow-up (figure 1.1). Available resources should be allocated efficiently among these, and within each of them, so as to achieve the maximum net improvement in health outcomes at whatever level of resource commitment is chosen.

The structuring of the problem is further illustrated by the state-transition model shown in figure 1.2. The ultimate aim is to move as many hypertensives as possible from their initial state—unaware, aware but not in care, or in care but uncontrolled—to a controlled state. Interventions available have different effects on this rightward flow in the diagram. Screening, for example, reduces the numbers of hypertensives who are unaware of their condition, while efforts to improve follow-up, including patient education, are designed to ensure that patients remain in care and ultimately have their blood pressures controlled. The effectiveness of any intervention is measured in terms of resultant changes in the distribution of individuals among states and consequent reductions in mortality and morbidity. Benefits are balanced against the costs associated with interventions and those of maintaining an individual in a given state.

The book is organized according to this analytic framework.

The basic analysis of the benefits, costs, and risks of treatment for hypertension is presented in chapter 2. This is then followed by a more detailed analysis of the issue of drug side effects and the impact of these on optimal treatment decisions (chapter 3). Chapter 4 introduces the problem of incomplete adherence as one of the obstacles that impede effective control of hypertension and analyzes the importance of adherence as a factor in determining the cost-effectiveness of treatment. After alternative screening strategies are assessed in chapter 5, a model for resource allocation decisions involving screening, referral, diagnosis, treatment, and follow-up is developed (chapter 6). Chapter 7 then evaluates the use of diagnostic procedures to detect secondary, or curable, hypertension. The final chapter summarizes the major findings of the analysis and presents a set of policy recommendations based on them.

2. Cost-Effectiveness of Treatment

This chapter assesses the components of cost and effectiveness associated with the medical treatment of hypertension, and thereby serves as the cornerstone for the analysis in subsequent chapters. These questions are addressed:

• Given the available data, and making alternative sets of assumptions about parameters for which data are lacking, to what extent is treatment of elevated blood pressure a cost-effective use of scarce health care resources?

• Given that available resources are limited, what groups of individuals—by sex, age, blood pressure level, race, or other risk factors—should be given highest priority for treatment?

• To what extent does treatment of high blood pressure "pay for itself" in that costs of treatment are recovered in expected savings from treating subsequent illness?

• To what extent do the side effects of therapy mitigate its benefits and render antihypertensive therapy an inappropriate use of resources?

• To which parameters are the above conclusions most sensitive, and what are the implications for research policy?

The current state of knowledge about hypertension provides the basis for this analysis. In areas where this knowledge is secure, conclusions can be reached with confidence. In areas where only partial information or subjective assessments are available, greater uncertainty exists, and conclusions must be coupled with the realization that they can and will be altered as new information is accumulated. Where uncertainty exists, the sensitivity of conclusions drawn to the parameters employed can be evaluated and critical areas requiring future research identified. The tendency among health professionals to demand objective, scien-

17

tifically valid proof, though laudable, begs the necessity to make current decisions. Difficult and unavoidable decisions are made daily by physicians and policy makers alike, frequently in the presence of considerable uncertainty. The important thing is to make the best possible decision given the current state of knowledge, for to wait until all the evidence is in constitutes a decision by default.

THE COST-EFFECTIVENESS CRITERION FOR RESOURCE ALLOCATION

The major objective of a hypertension treatment program, from the point of view of society, is to maximize benefits derived from a given net medical expenditure. The criterion for cost-effectiveness, therefore, is the ratio of the net increase in medical care costs to net effectiveness in terms of enhanced life expectancy and quality of life.

Net medical care costs must take into account:

• the incremental cost of a lifetime of antihypertensive treatment (ΔC_{Rx}),
• the savings of treatment costs resulting from reductions in the number of cardiovascular morbid events ($-\Delta C_{Morb}$),
• the costs of treating side effects of antihypertensive medication (ΔC_{SE}), and
• the costs of treating any noncardiovascular illnesses which occur in the added years of life expectancy conferred by treatment and which, therefore, would not have occurred in the absence of treatment ($\Delta C_{Rx \triangle LE}$).

Net health effectiveness, on the other hand, is measured in terms of increased years of life expectancy, adjusted to account for changes in the quality of life due to the prevention of morbid events and due to the side effects of antihypertensive therapy. It is measured here as the algebraic sum of:

• the increase in life expectancy resulting from adherence to a lifelong blood pressure lowering regimen (ΔY_{LE}),
• the value, in terms of an equivalently valued number of life years, of the increased capacity for work, activity, and improved quality of life that result from reduced cardiovascular morbidity (ΔY_{Morb}), and
• the value, in the same terms, of the net reduction in the

quality of life that results from antihypertensive treatment $(-\Delta Y_{SE})$. The inconvenience, anxiety, and pharmacologic side effects associated with medical regimens, as well as relief of symptoms attributable to untreated hypertension, are all considered.

While these components of health effectiveness might have been valued in dollar terms based on lost earnings or some other measure of cost, it is considered more appropriate to value health effects in health terms—life years—leaving the implicit tradeoff between costs and life years to society's decision-making agents.

The cost-effectiveness ratio based on these criteria,

$$\frac{C}{E} = \frac{\Delta C_{Rx} - \Delta C_{Morb} + \Delta C_{SE} + \Delta C_{Rx\triangle LE}}{\Delta Y_{LE} + \Delta Y_{Morb} - \Delta Y_{SE}}, \qquad (2.1)$$

provides the decision maker with an index by which to establish priorities for the allocation of limited resources. To maximize total benefits, resources should be allocated according to values of the C/E ratio for different classes of patients characterized by age, sex, blood pressure level, and other risk factors. The cutoff value of the ratio would be determined either by the limits of available resources or by an absolute value above which treatment was considered inefficient relative to other uses of the resources.

Decision makers involved in the actual delivery of care, including patients and providers, may apply different criteria in making their individual decisions, however, and thus depart from socially optimal rules for decision making. The differences between society's criterion, on the one hand, and those of the diverse individual decision makers, on the other, are of particular importance in analyzing factors involved in the implementation of cost-effective practices.

An individual patient who is fully covered by health insurance will not be concerned with cost. Such a patient will consider only the net health benefit of treatment, as given by the denominator of the ratio, and will elect treatment if and only if this net health benefit is positive. A patient who pays part or all of the medical bill will balance the net health benefit against the cost he must pay in making that choice. In either case, the resulting decision about therapy will not necessarily coincide with society's priorities based on cost-effectiveness. While the fully insured patient may not consider cost at all, the patient who must pay out of pocket may weigh the cost more heavily than would society. Moreover, the patient's perception of net health benefit may well differ from the medical assessment.

A fee-for-service physician may apply still other criteria. In representing the interests of each individual patient he may choose to initiate treatment whenever net health benefit is positive and to select the treatment that will maximize net health benefit regardless of cost. Alternatively, he may act in accordance with constraints on his time and give priority to patients according to the amount of provider time required per unit health benefit achieved (rather than total cost per health benefit). Moreover, he may, for personal or professional reasons, tend to favor procedures that yield special satisfaction: procedures that produce immediate dramatic results are often preferred to those requiring long-term care, irrespective of cost or cost-effectiveness. For these reasons and others, decisions made by fee-for-service physicians in their practices frequently depart from those indicated by socially optimal allocations of resources. This is true of allocations both within hypertension and between hypertension and other health problems.

Prepaid practices such as health maintenance organizations, in theory at least, apply criteria that coincide with those of society in seeking to maximize health benefits to their patient populations within limited budgets. Because they are composed of providers with similar educations and goals as fee-for-service physicians, however, some of the same biases persist and, in many instances, may override their greater emphasis on cost containment. Moreover, health maintenance organizations may tend to evaluate preventive medical care primarily in terms of cost. Preventive services that do not "pay for themselves" by avoiding more future medical costs than they entail may be viewed less favorably. Hence, though the objectives of health maintenance organizations do lead to concern for resource allocation, the criteria they apply to balance cost and benefit may still differ somewhat from those society as a whole would apply.

Because each of these decision makers applies different criteria, the medical care decisions that result cannot be expected to be in full accord with societal concerns. Nevertheless, resource allocation criteria based on maximizing net health benefit per dollar spent do provide a standard by which the performance of the health care system can be judged and a goal toward which it should move.

Methods

This overview of the methodology used to assess the cost-effectiveness of antihypertensive treatment highlights the major steps leading to the estimation of the cost-effectiveness ratio (equation 2.1). A more detailed description of the computational procedures used may be found in the appendix to this chapter.

DATA BASE FOR RISK REDUCTION

Data from the Framingham Heart Study [Kannel and Gordon, 1970, 1974] were utilized to assess the relationship between blood pressure and subsequent mortality and morbidity. Though that study does not provide direct information on the effectiveness of antihypertensive treatment, it is the single best source available which quantifies the longitudinal relationship between blood pressure and risk in a free-standing population. Our analysis focuses on diastolic blood pressures despite the existence of similar relationships for systolic pressures.

According to the statistical analyses of the Framingham Study (described more fully in the appendix to this chapter), blood pressure has a multiplicative, not additive, effect on mortality and the incidence of morbid events. As seen in figure 2.1, mortality not only increases with blood pressure but increases at an accelerating rate (that is, the higher the level of blood pressure, the greater the increase in risk for a given increase in blood pressure). This property suggests that reduction of blood pressure from higher levels should yield greater benefits than comparable intervals of reduction from lower levels. To estimate the degree of benefit, it was assumed that reduction of blood pressure confers some fraction of the benefit that one would expect from examining the schedules of risk associated with natural blood pressures in the Framingham Study.

The Veterans Administration Cooperative Study on Antihypertensive Agents [1967, 1970], which demonstrated beneficial effects of treatment on mortality and morbidity for persons with diastolic pressures in excess of 105 mm Hg, has become the cornerstone for policy recommendations by the National Heart and Lung Institute and the American Heart Association. Limitations of that study, however, militated against deriving quantitative estimates from it for this analysis. These relate primarily to the nature of the selection process employed. The study popula-

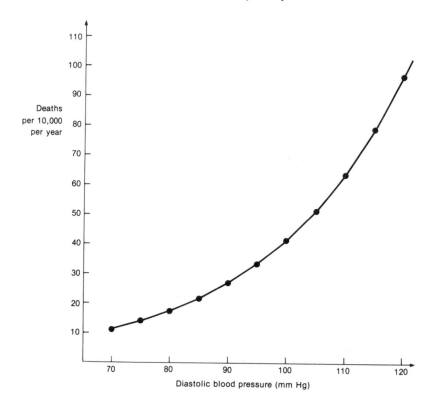

Figure 2.1: Risk function for mortality. This graph shows the annual mortality rate as a function of diastolic blood pressure for males 35–44 years of age, based on a statistical fitting of Framingham data to the "logistic" risk function. (Source: Framingham Heart Study [Kannel and Gordon, 1970].)

tion consisted solely of males with a mean age of 50 years, who voluntarily sought treatment, and who had a high prevalence of clinical symptoms or evidence of established vascular disease at the beginning of the study. Admission was limited to those whose diastolic pressures remained above 90 mm Hg after four to six days of hospitalization and was further limited to those who demonstrated their ability to comply with medical regimens. Hence study patients were unrepresentative of the general hypertensive population with respect to age, sex, severity of vascular disease, and ability to comply with medical regimens. Furthermore, because blood pressure measurements were taken in such a way as to ensure a basal state and to reduce measurement variability, it is difficult to equate the blood pressure levels for which beneficial results were obtained to those measured more casually in the general population.

Despite these limitations, however, the Veterans Administration Study does provide important qualitative evidence that blood pressure control does reduce risk. Without this evidence, the entire analysis would be based on mere speculation; with it, some confidence can be attached to the range of assumptions made describing the fraction of benefit achievable, at least for patients with moderate or severe hypertension.

BASIC ANALYTIC CONCEPTS EMPLOYED

Three fundamental concepts underlying the analysis deserve special discussion before turning to a description of the overall approach. These are (1) the estimation of the fraction of benefit achieved by treatment, (2) the concept of translating all effectiveness measures into quality-adjusted life years as a means for establishing common units for all measures of effectiveness, and (3) the principle of discounting applied to valuing future costs and benefits.

FRACTION OF BENEFIT.   To estimate the effect of blood pressure control on mortality and morbidity, it was recognized that an individual whose blood pressure is controlled from X to Y at age z does not necessarily become identical in risk to one whose natural blood pressure is Y at age z. Instead, it was assumed that the risk for such an individual is some weighted average of the risks corresponding to the controlled level and the level in the absence of control. This weight is termed the "fraction of benefit" (*FOB*). If *FOB* is 1.0, the risk is equal to that of the lower (controlled) blood pressure. This is the "full benefit assumption." If *FOB* is 0.0, the risk is equal to that of the higher (natural) blood pressure and no benefit is derived. If *FOB* is between 0.0 and 1.0, the risk is reduced by a fraction of the difference in risks between the two pressures. Figure 2.2 illustrates the use of fraction of benefit in a 40-year-old male whose diastolic blood pressure is reduced from 110 mm to 90 mm Hg. Under the full benefit assumption (*FOB* = 1.0), the risk of death is reduced from 64 to 27 per 10,000. If *FOB* is 0.5, the risk is reduced by only half the difference between the upper and lower bounds of risk, to 45.5 per 10,000. Finally, if *FOB* is 0.0, the risk of death associated with 110 mm Hg (64 per 10,000) still holds.

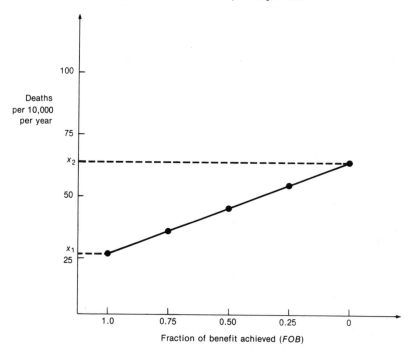

Figure 2.2: Use of fraction of benefit (*FOB*) in computing mortality rates. The effect of controlling diastolic blood pressure from 110 mm Hg to 90 mm Hg in a 40-year-old male is shown under different assumptions of fraction of benefit (*FOB*). *FOB* = 1.0 results in a mortality rate equivalent to that of an untreated diastolic blood pressure of 90 mm Hg (x_1); *FOB* = 0.0 results in a mortality rate equivalent to that of an untreated diastolic blood pressure of 110 mm Hg (x_2).

This concept is of particular importance for a condition such as hypertension with its long, predominantly asymptomatic, natural history, during which the time of diagnosis and initiation of treatment may be highly variable. An important consideration is that the fraction of benefit may not remain constant throughout the course of therapy but instead may increase directly with duration of blood pressure control due to prevention or reversal of cardiovascular disease. For similar reasons, the fraction of benefit is likely to depend upon the age at which blood pressure control is initiated, since the duration of blood pressure elevation prior to treatment is indicative of the extent of cumulative cardiovascular damage to that time. A sample set of subjective estimates of fraction of benefit as a function of age at initiation and duration

Table 2.1: Estimates of fraction of benefit (*FOB*) under the age-varying partial benefit assumption for mortality.

Duration of therapy (years)	Age at initiation of therapy				
	20	30	40	50	60
0–5	0.8	0.5	0.35	0.25	0.15
5–15	.85	.7	.6	.45	.3
15+	.9	.8	.7	.55	.4

of therapy is given in table 2.1 for mortality and in table 2.2 for strokes and myocardial infarctions. These provided the basis for the "age-varying partial benefit assumption," in contrast to the "full benefit assumption" ($FOB = 1.0$), the "half benefit assumption" ($FOB = 0.5$), and the "no benefit assumption" ($FOB = 0.0$), all of which are independent of age and duration of therapy. The full benefit assumption, in effect, asserts that the Framingham risk data are valid as predictors of the effects of blood pressure control, while all other assumptions indicate that they provide upper bounds only.

Estimates underlying the age-varying partial benefit assumption are, of necessity, subjective and are derived from evidence of the demonstrated effectiveness of antihypertensive treatment in preventing cerebral hemorrhages and malignant hypertension, and from suggestive evidence that it prevents or slows progression of the atherosclerotic vascular changes associated with hypertension. If these premises are valid, the degree of benefit would depend significantly on the age of the patient, the duration of the elevated blood pressure, and the condition of the vascular

Table 2.2: Estimates of fraction of benefit (*FOB*) under the age-varying partial benefit assumption for cerebrovascular accident and myocardial infarction.

Duration of therapy (years)	Age at initiation of therapy				
	20	30	40	50	60
Cerebrovascular accident					
0–5	0.9	0.75	0.68	0.62	0.57
5–15	.92	.85	.8	.72	.65
15+	.95	.9	.85	.78	.7
Myocardial infarction					
0–5	.4	.25	.18	.13	.08
5–15	.43	.35	.3	.23	.15
15+	.45	.4	.35	.28	.2

system at the time treatment was begun. The assumption thus favors treatment of younger patients. It remains to be proven, however, whether such is actually the case.

A "probabilistic benefit assumption" was also constructed to reflect the basic uncertainty that exists with regard to the true fraction of benefit to be derived from treatment. Under such uncertainty the decision process must take into account relative strengths of belief in the different assumptions considered. The example used in the analysis depicts a decision maker who believes there is a 40 percent likelihood that full benefit is true, a 40 percent likelihood that the configuration of age-varying partial benefit is true, and a 20 percent likelihood that no benefit occurs. Variants of this assumption can reflect any combination of subjective probabilities.

QUALITY-ADJUSTED LIFE YEARS. The second fundamental methodological principle employed stems from the necessity to translate all measures of effectiveness into common units, be they added years of life expectancy, enhanced quality of life resulting from prevention of morbid events, or the side effects associated with drug treatments. "Quality-adjusted life years" have been chosen as this measure.[1] For a patient dying suddenly, following a life unencumbered by morbidity from myocardial infarctions or cerebrovascular accidents, there is no problem. The measure of effectiveness is simply the number of added years of life expectancy conferred by treatment. For the individual who suffers a morbid event, does not die, but is subsequently disabled, there arises the necessity to quantify his altered quality of life. To do so the tradeoff between life years and disability is assessed by evaluating responses to the question: "Taking into account your pain and suffering, immobility, and lost earnings, what fraction of a year of life would you be willing to give up in order to have good health for the remaining fraction of a year instead of your present level of disability for the full year?" An answer near 1.0 implies that the level of disability is equivalent to death; an answer near 0.0, on the other hand, implies a mild or negligible level of disability. The basic tradeoff is disability for life years at

---

1. A similar measure was employed by Torrance, Sackett, and Thomas [1973] in their analysis of renal dialysis and tuberculosis programs and by Pliskin and Beck [1976] in their analysis of the choice between renal dialysis and transplantation. The methodological basis for this approach has been explored by Fanshel and Bush [1970]; Bush, Chen, and Patrick [1973]; Berg [1973]; and Forst [1973].

a given point in time. Similar considerations apply to the valuation of the side effects of therapy. For disability resulting from both morbid events and side effects, discounting corrects for the fact that it is often future years of life that are being traded for changes in the present quality of life.

This tradeoff concept is a difficult one. It is a very real one, however, and is faced daily, either explicitly or implicitly, by both providers and patients as they make health care decisions.

DISCOUNTING. A process intrinsic to all economic analyses, discounting takes into account the fact that dollars spent in the present are worth more than those spent in the future, the difference being, fundamentally, the rate of interest that present dollars would earn if they were invested rather than spent. Equivalently, future costs need to be deflated by an annual rate of discount corresponding to the real rate of return obtainable on invested dollars. The annual discount rate employed in this study was chosen to be 5 percent. Thus a cost of $1,000 incurred 10 years in the future is considered to have a present value of $1,000/$(1.05)^{10} \cong \$610$. The choice of an appropriate discount rate is a matter of some controversy among economists, but 5 percent approximates the real, after-tax rate of return acceptable to private investors in normal economic times,[2] and represents a compromise among the various economic schools of thought on this issue.

The discounting principle was also extended to life years to account for the fact that present years of life are generally valued more highly in present dollars than future years.[3] "Net present value" of quality-adjusted life expectancy was therefore computed by assigning to each year in the future a value relative to that of a year of life in the present. For example, if treatment is begun at age 40, the 40th year is valued as 1, the 41st year, conditional

---

2. Recently, recession and inflation have combined to make this rate of return somewhat lower, perhaps near zero. Historically, the real rate of return has been significantly higher.

3. Equivalently, it is more costly to spend a given number of dollars now to save a year of life in the future than to spend the same number of dollars in the future. Consider, for example, two programs. Program A costs $20,000 and, if spent by a 40-year-old, will save his 60th year. Program B costs $20,000 and, if spent by a 50-year-old, will save his 60th year. Program B is preferable for the following reason: if, instead of spending the $20,000 for program A, the 40-year-old invested the money to grow at 5 percent, at age 50 he would have $32,600—$(1.05)^{10} \times \$20,000$—and could then purchase program B and have $12,600 left over for other purposes.

upon survival, as $1/(1.05) \cong 0.95$, the 42nd year as $1/(1.05)^2$ $\cong 0.91$, and so forth.

Furthermore, it was assumed that a year of life at any age is worth the same as a year of life at any other age. Hence the 70th year is worth just as much to a 65-year-old as the 40th year is to a 35-year-old, but the 70th year is worth only $(1.05)^{-30}$ times as many present dollars as the 40th year is to a 35-year-old only because it is 30 years further into the future.[4]

The effect of discounting is to attach higher values to treatment costs and medication side effects in early years of life and to reductions in near-term morbidity and mortality, while attaching relatively lower values to distant life-years, reduced long-term morbidity, and future cost savings. For hypertension, it is obvious that treatment costs and medication side effects begin soon after the initiation of treatment, while morbid and mortal events occur largely in future years. Hence, discounting tends to mitigate the cost-effectiveness of early treatment.

CALCULATION OF COST-EFFECTIVENESS

Figure 2.3 presents an overview of the major steps involved in deriving the components of the cost-effectiveness ratio (equation 2.1). The steps leading to them are described briefly here and in more detail in the appendix to this chapter. Complete adherence to prescribed medical regimens is assumed throughout the analysis in this chapter. (The effects of incomplete adherence are considered in chapter 4.)

CATEGORIES OF PATIENTS ANALYZED. Patient categories were defined according to sex, age, pretreatment diastolic blood pressure, and achieved diastolic blood pressure. Both males and females were considered. Ages analyzed were 20 years (representing the decade 15–24), 30 years (25–34), 40 years (35–44), 50 years (45–54), and 60 years (55–64). Pretreatment blood pressures were chosen at 10 mm Hg intervals as follows: 90 mm Hg (representing the range 85–94 mm Hg), 100 mm Hg (95–104

---

4. Alternatively, the assumption might have been made that successive years in life are worth absolutely less in the sense that their quality deteriorates as more illness and disability develop with age. On the other hand, controlling for disability, later years could be considered to be worth *more* than younger years because of the wisdom, productivity, or freedom of responsibility that may accompany them. For purposes of this analysis, these effects were assumed to cancel, so that only pure discounting (or preference for present over future) applies.

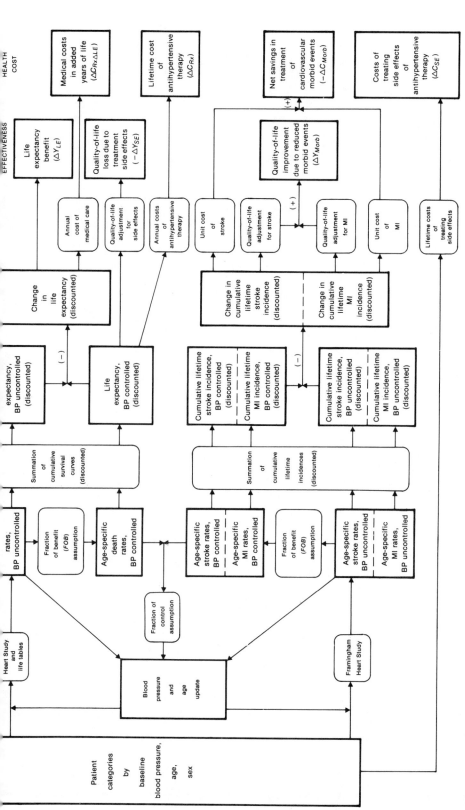

Figure 2.3: Diagrammatic summary of methods for assessing cost-effectiveness. This chart shows the major steps involved in deriving the components of the cost-effectiveness ratio $R = (\Delta Y_{LE} + \Delta Y_{Morb} - \Delta Y_{SE})/(\Delta C_{Rx} - \Delta C_{Morb} + \Delta C_{SE} + \Delta C_{Rx\Delta LE})$. Rounded boxes indicate places where data or assumptions were used.

mm Hg), 110 mm Hg (105–114 mm Hg), and 120 mm Hg
(115–124 mm Hg).

Two alternative assumptions were made regarding the degree
of blood pressure control achieved. The first of these holds that
a patient whose blood pressure is above 90 mm Hg is controlled
to 90 mm Hg, regardless of the initial level. The second and
probably more realistic assumption postulates a stepped schedule
of blood pressure reduction, such that the higher the initial level
of blood pressure the greater the decrement attained yet the
higher the controlled level. The latter, called the "stepped control"
assumption, can be thought of as reflecting the average degrees
of control clinically achievable within an acceptable range of
medication side effects. The stepped control assumption is summarized in table 2.3.

ESTIMATION OF MORTALITY RATES AND LIFE EXPECTANCY.
Calculation of anticipated increased life expectancy due to antihypertensive treatment involved three steps:

• estimation of mortality rates as functions of age, sex, and
blood pressure levels,
• computation of life expectancy for patients whose blood
pressures are not being medically controlled, and
• computation of increases in life expectancy for patients whose
blood pressures are being controlled medically, based upon various degrees of control achieved and on the concept that treatment confers some fraction of the benefit implied by the schedule
of risk associated with natural blood pressure.

The Framingham Heart Study [Kannel and Gordon, 1970,
1974] provided the relationship between uncontrolled diastolic
blood pressure and mortality for each decade between ages 35
and 74 and for both sexes. The Framingham Study's risk estimates were adjusted upward using standard life tables [National

Table 2.3: **Blood pressure control achieved under the stepped control
assumption.**

Uncontrolled diastolic blood pressure (mm Hg)	Stepped control diastolic blood pressure (mm Hg)
90	80
100	85
110	90
120	95

Center for Health Statistics, 1968] to account for the fact that the population cohort was healthier than the general population, by virtue of being composed largely of individuals with no prior evidence of cardiovascular abnormalities. Risk estimates were extrapolated to age groups younger (18–34) and older (75 and above) than those included in the Framingham Study. The details of both of these procedures, and of other assumptions underlying the use of the Framingham data, are described in the appendix to this chapter.

The fraction of benefit procedure described previously was used to derive mortality rates for the patient under blood pressure control as a weighted average of the Framingham rates at the uncontrolled and controlled levels (see figure 2.2). Table 2.1 gives the parameters of the age-varying partial benefit assumption for mortality used in the analysis.

The natural rise of blood pressure with age was derived from national data [National Center for Health Statistics, 1964a]. (See the appendix to this chapter.) For the patient under blood pressure control, however, it was assumed that only a fraction of the natural rise could be controlled by therapy within tolerable levels of medication side effects. This fraction of control (*FC*) was arbitrarily set at 0.5 for the present analysis. Thus, if the uncontrolled diastolic blood pressure would have risen by 5 mm Hg per decade, then the controlled diastolic blood pressure was assumed to rise by 2.5 mm Hg per decade. The effect of this parameter on the rise of blood pressure with age is illustrated in figure 2.4.

To calculate life expectancy, survival curves (that is, schedules of annual mortality rates) were generated for each patient category. Life expectancies were computed by the standard method of summation of cumulative survival curves, except that the principle of discounting future life years was applied as described previously. The differences between life expectancies, discounted, for the uncontrolled and controlled patients were then derived. This difference is the term ΔY_{LE} in the denominator of the cost-effectiveness ratio (equation 2.1).

ESTIMATION OF THE LIFETIME COST OF ANTIHYPERTENSIVE TREATMENT. Costs of treating high blood pressure include those of medications, physician visits, and laboratory examinations. Since retail prices vary widely, average costs of medications were estimated by doubling the wholesale drug prices to retailers

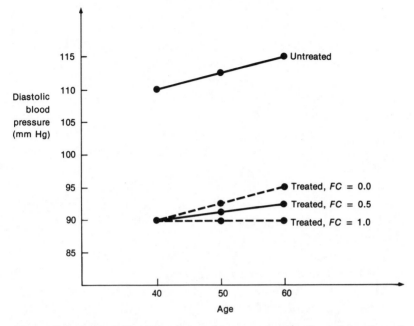

Figure 2.4: Rise of blood pressure with age as a function of control (FC). The incremental rise in diastolic blood pressure with age, 2.5 mm Hg per decade, is depicted under various assumptions regarding the ability of antihypertensive treatment to control this increment. The example is for a male whose blood pressure at age 40 was 110 mm Hg, reduced initially by treatment to 90 mm Hg.

for regimens commonly employed in the treatment of mild to moderate essential hypertension. These are summarized in table 2.4. Costs vary widely depending on the drug regimen used. To medication costs are added those incurred by physician visits that can be directly attributed to the treatment of hypertension, estimated at the equivalent of three visits costing $10 to $15 per visit, and annual costs of laboratory tests, estimated at about $20 to $30. Thus the total annual cost ranges from $133 to $403. An average value of $200 was used in this analysis, reflecting the fact that less expensive regimens are more commonly prescribed. To this cost was added a first year diagnostic work-up cost of $100. Discounted treatment costs were computed as the net present value of the stream of costs over the expected lifetime, and compose the term ΔC_{Rx} in the numerator of the cost-effectiveness ratio (equation 2.1).

ESTIMATION OF THE INCIDENCE OF MORBID EVENTS.   Reductions in the expected numbers of cerebrovascular accidents and

Table 2.4: Yearly costs of common antihypertensive drug regimens.

Drug regimen	Yearly cost
Diuretic only	$ 83
Diuretic and reserpine	112
Diuretic and alpha-methyldopa	180
Diuretic, hydralazine, and propranolol	328

Figures are based on doubling prices paid by retailers [*Drug Topics Red Book,* 1975]. Assumed doses are: chlorothiazide (diuretic) 1,000 mg/day; reserpine 0.25 mg/day; alpha-methyldopa 500 mg/day; hydralazine 100 mg/day; and propranolol 160 mg/day.

myocardial infarctions enter the cost-effectiveness calculation in two ways. First, they represent savings in medical costs (constituting the term ΔC_{Morb}). Second, they reflect improvements in quality of life, measured here in terms of equivalently valued numbers of life years (constituting the term ΔY_{Morb}).

Expected changes in the numbers of cerebrovascular accidents and myocardial infarctions were computed by methods comparable to those used to compute increase in life expectancy. Other complications associated with sustained hypertension, such as congestive heart failure, dissecting aortic aneurysm, and renal damage were not considered, because they are substantially less important than stroke and heart attack in terms of overall morbidity and cost.

The Framingham Heart Study provided data on the risk of morbid events. Incidence rates for individuals under blood pressure control were calculated under alternative fraction of benefit assumptions. The age-varying partial benefit assumption (table 2.2) reflects the substantially greater fractional benefit for stroke than for myocardial infarction that was demonstrated in the Veterans Administration Study [1967, 1970]. The methods used to estimate changes in the expected lifetime incidence of morbid events are described in detail in the appendix to this chapter.

VALUATION OF IMPROVEMENT IN QUALITY OF LIFE FROM RE-DUCED CARDIOVASCULAR MORBIDITY.   The prevention of a morbid event has value to the individual patient not only in terms of prolonged life but also in terms of increased ability to work and improved quality of life. This benefit might be valued in dollar terms as a cost savings to society (as distinguished from the actual savings of medical care costs considered separately), but it is more natural to value it in terms that are meaningful to the individual patient. To do so, this analysis attempts to translate any given level of morbidity or disability into quality-adjusted life years as described previously.

For stroke, results of a study by Emlet et al. [1973] were used to provide estimates of disability. In that study, a panel of experts assessed, for each of four classes of stroke victims, the expected number of years to be spent in each of several disability states following a first stroke. Thus, the morbid effects of all recurrences are taken into account. These estimates were supplemented by our own estimates of disability for the remaining stroke victims who are mildly affected or who die. Each level of disability was assigned a life-years equivalent, ranging from 0.9 years of life lost per year of total dependency to 0.05 years of life lost per year of mild residual symptoms. The value of future years of disability was discounted appropriately to give present-value estimates. The details of this analysis, and the data upon which it is based, are given in the appendix to this chapter. The result was an expected quality loss of 1.5 present-value life-year equivalents per incident stroke.

For myocardial infarction, both the frequency and relative severity of residual disability are markedly less than for strokes. The analysis, based on identical methods but using entirely subjective data, is described in the appendix to this chapter. An estimate of 0.5 present-value life-year equivalents lost per incident myocardial infarction was derived.

The expected increase in (discounted) quality-adjusted life expectancy due to the prevention of morbid events was calculated by multiplying the (discounted) change in lifetime incidence for each type of event by the respective life-year equivalents of morbidity (1.5 years for stroke and 0.5 years for myocardial infarction). The sum becomes the estimate of ΔY_{Morb} in the denominator of the cost-effectiveness ratio.

ESTIMATION OF COST SAVINGS FROM CARDIOVASCULAR MORBIDITY PREVENTED.   For stroke the results of the study by Emlet et al. [1973] were utilized. In that study, the total present value of medical and rehabilitation costs of treating the initial event and any recurrences was estimated for the categories of patients to which these data applied. For patients who die during the initial episode and for those who do not suffer significant residual disability, independent estimates of cost were made. An average present-value cost saved per initial stroke prevented was computed to be about $10,000 (see the appendix to this chapter). For myocardial infarction, costs were estimated using Medicare data for hospital care [Social Security Administration, 1974a] and independent estimates for subsequent ambulatory care. The Medicare data may overestimate true hospital cost because length of stay tends to increase with age, but this is not a serious limitation since the importance of myocardial infarction costs in the analysis is found to be minimal. Probabilities of recurrences were estimated explicitly using a branching model based on the medical literature and subjective estimates. The analysis, described in the appendix to this chapter, resulted in a present-value estimate of $7,000 in medical costs per initial myocardial infarction prevented.

To compute the net (discounted) cost savings from prevention of cerebrovascular accidents and myocardial infarctions, the (discounted) changes in the lifetime probabilities of each were multiplied by their respective unit costs. The sum was then used as an estimate of ΔC_{Morb} in the numerator of the cost-effectiveness ratio.

VALUATION OF IMPAIRMENT OF QUALITY OF LIFE DUE TO TREATMENT SIDE EFFECTS. The final component of the net effectiveness of antihypertensive therapy is the net influence of the therapeutic regimen on quality of life. Though difficult to quantify, it is essential to do so, however imperfectly, in any comprehensive assessment of the net benefits of treatment. For hypertension, which is asymptomatic in the large majority of cases, this is particularly important because future benefits may have to be traded for near-term impairment in the quality of life.

Except for the possible relationship of treatment with reserpine to breast cancer, increases in mortality caused by commonly used antihypertensive drugs are very small relative to the reductions achieved by blood pressure control. In the present analysis, therefore, drug-induced mortality was assumed to be zero. The sensitivity of the results to that assumption is tested in chapter 3, where a full discussion of side effects is given.

The effects of a therapeutic regimen on the quality of life include the value of any symptomatic relief it provides, the inconvenience it imposes, and the side effects of the medications. The latter are frequent and vary in severity from mild drowsiness and excessive urination to depression and impotence. Because hypertension is usually asymptomatic, the overall effect is typically negative.

Since no empirical means is available to assess these subjective costs to the patient, a single parameter was employed, reflecting the fraction of one's life one would be willing to sacrifice in order to avoid them. In this analysis, a value of .01 was chosen arbitrarily, reflecting a willingness to give up about four days out of each year in exchange for relief from side effects. Multiplying total (or discounted) life expectancy by this fraction, the final term (ΔY_{SE}) in the denominator of the cost-effectiveness ratio was estimated.

ESTIMATION OF THE COSTS OF TREATING MEDICATION SIDE EFFECTS. Present-value expected lifetime costs of treating severe drug complications such as depression, ulcer, and gout are estimated to average about $125 per patient receiving antihypertensive treatment (see chapter 3).

ESTIMATION OF MEDICAL COSTS INCURRED IN THE ADDED YEARS OF LIFE EXPECTANCY. Often ignored are the costs of medical care received during extended years of life. Credit given to control of blood pressure for reducing costs associated with treatment of strokes and myocardial infarctions must be balanced against medical costs for other diseases incurred during the added years of life [Thorner, 1970]. An estimate of $300 annually was made for these costs, based on the estimated national per capita expenditure of about $400 per year for persons 55 and older, of which 75 percent was assumed to be for treatment of other than cardiovascular diseases [Health Resources Administration, 1973]. Total costs were then computed to be the increase in discounted life expectancy in years (ΔY_{LE}) times $300.

COMPUTATION OF THE NET COST OF ANTIHYPERTENSIVE TREATMENT

A number of health care decision makers, including the managers of health insurance programs and health maintenance organizations, may have interest in knowing the extent to which a high blood pressure control program would "pay for itself" in terms of the strokes and heart attacks that otherwise would have required treatment. To that end, the average percentage of gross treatment costs that can be recovered from savings in the treatment of strokes and heart attacks was calculated for United

States adults with diastolic blood pressures of 105 mm Hg or above. This calculation was made by applying to the 1975 adult population by age [Social Security Administration, 1974b] the estimated prevalences of blood pressures in the ranges 105–114 mm Hg and over 115 mm Hg [National Center for Health Statistics, 1964a] to estimate the number of men and women in each age and blood pressure class. These numbers were multiplied by the estimated expected lifetime treatment costs (ΔC_{Rx}) and summed to give gross costs. They were then multiplied by the estimated expected cost savings from cardiovascular morbidity prevented (ΔC_{Morb}) and summed to give total savings due to prevention of strokes and myocardial infarctions. The ratio of the latter to the former gives a sense of the extent to which the costs of antihypertensive therapy can be recouped. The costs of treating side effects were omitted from this calculation.

COMPUTATION OF THE AGGREGATE NATIONAL COST-EFFECTIVENESS OF ANTIHYPERTENSIVE TREATMENT

To combine the cost-effectiveness results by age, sex, and pretreatment diastolic blood pressure into a single quantity, the aggregate national cost-effectiveness of antihypertensive treatment was calculated. Two aggregate ratios were computed, one for persons with moderate and severe hypertension (diastolic blood pressures of 105 mm Hg and above) and one for persons with mild hypertension (diastolic blood pressures between 95 mm Hg and 105 mm Hg). The numerator of the aggregate cost-effectiveness ratio was calculated by multiplying the prevalence of each age, sex, and blood pressure category treated [Social Security Administration, 1974b; National Center for Health Statistics, 1964a] by the corresponding net lifetime treatment cost (the numerator in equation 2.1) and adding these together. The denominator was calculated by multiplying these same prevalences by the corresponding net increase in quality-adjusted life expectancy (the denominator in equation 2.1) and summing these. The resulting ratios give an overview of the estimated cost-effectiveness of antihypertensive treatment in the United States adult population.

SENSITIVITY ANALYSIS

Table 2.5 summarizes the parameter values and quantitative assumptions used in the analysis. Since most of these are based

Table 2.5: Summary of assumptions used in the analysis.

Parameter	Values used	Sources
Coefficients of risk function for mortality and morbidity	Framingham estimates for 18-year follow-up; extrapolations to ages <35 using 35–44 values; extrapolation to ages >74 using 65–74 values	Framingham Heart Study [Kannel and Gordon, 1970, 1974]
Base mortality rates	Life table values	Life tables, New England region [National Center for Health Statistics, 1968]
Slope of blood pressure change with age	1. Unadjusted natural history assumption	1. NHES cross-sectional data [National Center for Health Statistics, 1964a]
	2. Adjusted natural history assumption	2. NHES cross-sectional data adjusted for selective mortality [National Center for Health Statistics, 1964a]
Fractions of benefit for mortality and morbidity[a]	1. Full benefit assumption ($FOB = 1.0$)	1. Upper bound
	2. Half benefit assumption ($FOB = 0.5$)	2. Arbitrary
	3. Age-varying partial benefit (tables 2.1, 2.2)	3. Subjective estimates
	4. Probabilistic benefit (0.4 chance of full benefit, 0.4 chance of age-varying partial benefit, 0.2 chance of no benefit)	4. Subjective estimates
Degree of blood pressure control achieved[a]	1. Control to 90 mm Hg	1. Goal pressure cited by the National High Blood Pressure Education Program [1973b]
	2. Stepped control 120 to 95 mm Hg 110 to 90 mm Hg 100 to 85 mm Hg 90 to 80 mm Hg	2. Subjective assessment of commonly achieved levels with full adherence to drug regimen
Fraction of control for increments of blood pressure with age	0.5	Subjective estimate
Discount rate[a]	1. Undiscounted	1. Lower bound
	2. 5% per annum	2. Social rate of time preference
	3. 10% per annum	3. Upper bound

Table 2.5 (continued).

Parameter	Values used	Sources
Treatment cost[a]	$200 per year (range: $100–$300 per year) + $100 in the first year	Drug prices, physician charges, and laboratory costs as estimated in chapter 3
Medical cost per incident stroke[a]	$10,000 (range: $7,000–$15,000)	Emlet et al. [1973] and subjective estimates
Medical cost per incident MI[a]	$7,000 (range: $5,000–$10,000)	Medicare data [Social Security Administration, 1974a] and subjective estimates
Equivalent life-year loss per incident stroke[a]	1.5 years (range: 1.0–2.0 years)	Emlet et al. [1973] and subjective estimates
Equivalent life-year loss per incident MI[a]	0.5 years (range: 0.4–1.0 years)	Subjective estimates
Expected lifetime cost of treating complications of therapy	$125 (present value at 5% per annum)	Chapter 3
Expected annual cost of noncardiovascular medical care in added years of life	$300	HEW data [Health Resources Administration, 1973]
Equivalent life-year cost of side effects[a]	0.01 × life expectancy (range: [0.0–0.05] × life expectancy)	Subjective estimates

[a] Denotes parameters for which explicit sensitivity analyses were conducted.

on uncertain or subjective data, analysis was performed to determine the effect on results of perturbations in parameter values. The degree of sensitivity to changes in a given variable provides a measure of the level of confidence that one can have in the results and indicates areas to which efforts should be directed to obtain more precise estimates. Parameters for which sensitivity analysis was explicitly conducted were: fraction of benefit, degree of blood pressure control achieved, the discount rate, medical treatment costs, medical costs of strokes and myocardial infarctions, equivalent life-year losses for incident strokes and myocardial infarctions, and equivalent life-year losses due to treatment side effects.

Results

The cost-effectiveness of treatment, measured as the net lifetime medical cost per quality-adjusted year of life saved, was found to vary according to patient characteristics and according to the fraction of benefit assumption employed. The relationships between cost-effectiveness and blood pressure level, age, and sex, presented in the following section, lead to priorities for treatment and criteria for resource allocation. A sensitivity analysis reveals where these conclusions depend most heavily on key assumptions and suggests areas for future research.

To gain a sense of perspective on the magnitude of the benefit of treatment, increases in life expectancy were estimated. These are shown in table 2.6 for a reduction of diastolic blood pressure from 110 mm Hg to 90 mm Hg, without discounting and assuming full benefit. The increase in life expectancy ranges from 1.4 years for a 60-year-old male to 8.1 years for a 20-year-old male. Females of all age groups have intermediate values. Hence, the impact of treatment on survival is potentially considerable.

RELATIONSHIP OF COST-EFFECTIVENESS OF TREATMENT TO AGE AND SEX

The effect of age on cost-effectiveness is multifaceted. If treatment early in life prevents or retards the progression of the atherosclerotic vascular changes as postulated under the age-varying partial benefit assumption, effectiveness measures are markedly enhanced in younger age groups. These are balanced, however, by the greater costs incurred by longer periods of therapy, the increased duration of medication side effects, and

Table 2.6: Increase in life expectancy due to antihypertensive treatment, by age and sex.

Age	Life expectancy (years)	Increase in life expectancy (years) with treatment
Males		
20	46.5	8.1
30	38.2	5.8
40	29.7	3.9
50	21.7	2.5
60	14.8	1.4
Females		
20	53.2	5.0
30	43.9	4.4
40	34.8	3.7
50	26.4	2.8
60	18.5	2.3

Estimates exclude side effects and adjustments for morbidity and are for a reduction in diastolic blood pressure from 110 mm Hg to 90 mm Hg. Assumes: full benefit; no discounting.

the greater impact of discounting future benefits relative to present costs. For older individuals, mirror images of these arguments apply. Atherosclerotic vascular damage is more likely to be established by the time antihypertensive treatment is begun, and hence the expected fraction of benefit is less. At the same time, however, the lifetime cost of therapy is less, side effects operate over shorter periods of time, and discounting has relatively less effect both because of the shorter duration of therapy and because the mortal and morbid events prevented are more proximate.

Age when therapy is begun is important for an additional reason as well. Coefficients of risk for hypertension, calculated from the Framingham Heart Study, are larger for young than for old individuals. Hence, the *relative* risk conferred by hypertension decreases with increasing age. Since older people have higher overall mortality rates, however, the *absolute* risk conferred appears to increase with age. The number of life years saved per death averted is greater in younger people, however, so that on balance the increase in life expectancy for a given change in blood pressure, even assuming age-constant benefit, decreases with age (table 2.6).

Figure 2.5 displays the cost per year of life saved as a function of age at initiation of therapy with and without the application of discounting at 5 percent per annum. Results are for a reduction of diastolic blood pressure from 110 mm Hg to 90 mm Hg. The age-varying partial benefit assumption is employed, and all costs and effects are included as given by the cost-effectiveness ratio (equation 2.1).

The net cost per year of increased quality-adjusted life expectancy, with discounting, ranges from about $3,300 for 20-year-old males to $16,300 for 60-year-old males, and from about $8,500 for 20-year-old females down to about $5,000 for 60-year-old females. Thus, it appears to be relatively more cost-effective to treat men at earlier ages than women and to treat older women than older men. The crossing point is between ages 40 and 50. One explanation for this is the fact that atherosclerotic complications occur later in life in women than in men. As will be shown, these results for sex differences are robust and very unlikely to be affected by uncertainties underlying any of the assumptions upon which the analysis is based.

Discounting is seen to roughly double the costs per year of life

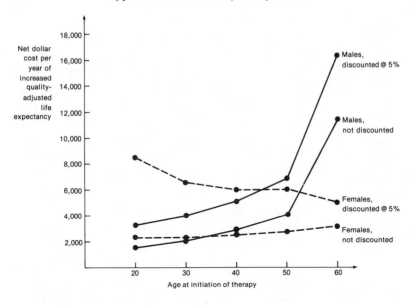

Figure 2.5: Cost-effectiveness by sex and by age at initiation of treatment. Results are given by age and sex, with and without discounting at 5 percent per annum, for a reduction in diastolic blood pressure from 110 mm Hg to 90 mm Hg. Assumes: age-varying partial benefit; complete adherence to medical regimens.

saved relative to not discounting, emphasizing the fact that the years of life saved occur mainly in the distant future while the costs of treatment occur throughout life. As expected, these effects are more pronounced in younger age groups.

RELATIONSHIP OF COST-EFFECTIVENESS OF TREATMENT TO THE FRACTION OF BENEFIT ASSUMPTION CHOSEN

Cost-effectiveness estimates are sensitive to which fraction of benefit assumption is chosen. Figures 2.6 and 2.7 compare, for males and females respectively, cost-effectiveness under the various fraction of benefit assumptions for an individual whose diastolic blood pressure is reduced from 110 mm Hg to 90 mm Hg. Discounting was employed, as it is in all subsequent results.

If antihypertensive treatment reduces the risk of mortality to that of nonhypertensive individuals of similar age and sex (full benefit assumption), then the cost per year of life saved is around $2,500 for men in all age groups. For women, however, treatment begun later in life is markedly more cost-effective than when begun earlier, a result related to the later occurrence of

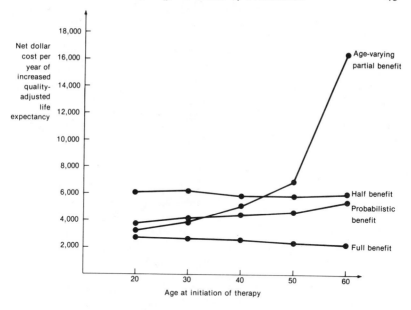

Figure 2.6: Effect of fraction of benefit assumption on cost-effectiveness of treatment for males. Results are given by age at initiation of treatment for a reduction in diastolic blood pressure from 110 mm Hg to 90 mm Hg. Probabilistic benefit indicates a 40 percent chance that full benefit holds, 40 percent chance that age-varying partial benefit holds, 20 percent chance that no benefit holds. Assumes: discounting at 5 percent per annum; complete adherence to medical regimens.

morbid events in women. Full benefit cost-effectiveness for women ranges from $7,700 per year of life saved at age 20 to only $1,800 at age 60.

The effect of the half benefit assumption is to more than double the estimates for full benefit in all age groups, but without changing the observed age trends. For younger women, this difference is especially dramatic because the importance of side effects increases, relative to the reduced benefits attributed to therapy.

The age-varying partial benefit assumption, because it assigns a higher fraction of benefit to treatment in younger age groups, makes early treatment relatively more cost-effective. This is particularly striking in men, in whom the cost per year of life saved ranges from $3,300 for a 20-year-old to $16,300 for a 60-year-old. For women, the age trend seen under the full benefit assumption is still evident, though with a reduced slope, and the resultant cost-effectiveness ratio falls from around $8,500 per year of life saved at age 20 to around $5,000 at age 60.

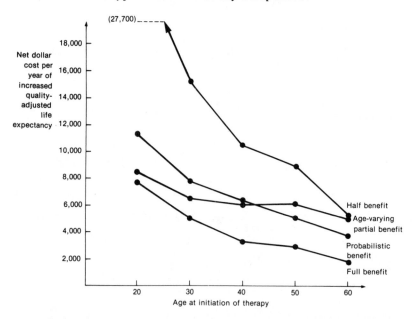

Figure 2.7: Effect of fraction of benefit assumption on cost-effectiveness of treatment for females. Results are given by age at initiation of treatment for a reduction in diastolic blood pressure from 110 mm Hg to 90 mm Hg. Probabilistic benefit indicates a 40 percent chance that full benefit holds, 40 percent chance that age-varying partial benefit holds, 20 percent chance that no benefit holds. Assumes: discounting at 5 percent per annum; complete adherence to medical regimens.

The probabilistic benefit assumption, which derives from the basic uncertainty of the true degree of benefit conferred by treatment, results in estimates largely intermediate between those of full benefit and partial benefit. In the younger age groups, however, the age-varying partial benefit assumption is close enough to the full benefit assumption that even a 20 percent probability of no benefit pulls the cost per year saved above that for partial benefit. The assignment of these particular probabilities to each fraction of benefit assumption is merely illustrative. A decision maker can incorporate whatever set of probabilities he wishes for full, half, age-varying, and no benefit to derive cost-effectiveness estimates consistent with his own beliefs.

RELATIONSHIP OF COST-EFFECTIVENESS OF TREATMENT TO BLOOD PRESSURE LEVEL

Both pretreatment and posttreatment blood pressures critically influence the cost-effectiveness ratio. Pretreatment blood pressure does so in several ways. First, because of the curvilinear nature of the risk relationship, equal decrements in blood pressure from higher levels result in greater absolute reductions in mortality and morbidity than from lower levels. When viewed in terms of life expectancy, however, this effect is mitigated somewhat because people with lower pressures have longer life expectancies to start with, so that any given relative change in their annual mortality rates would cause a greater absolute change in life expectancy than would an equal change for people with shorter life expectancies.[5] Second, the pretreatment blood pressure level influences the absolute degree of blood pressure control that is achievable. The higher the initial pressure, the greater the expected decrement in pressure, but also the higher the final pressure is likely to be. It is, on average, more difficult to control a patient from 120 mm Hg to 90 mm Hg than from 100 mm Hg to 90 mm Hg. This reality is taken into account in the stepped control assumption (table 2.3). Likewise, blood pressure may become more difficult to control with increasing age of the patient. The fraction of control parameter attempts to adjust for this fact by assuming that only half of the increase in blood pressure that occurs with increase in age is amenable to treatment within tolerable limits of medication side effects.

Figure 2.8 displays the cost per year of life saved as a function of pretreatment blood pressure under two assumptions of the degree of control achieved: control to 90 mm Hg or according to the stepped control schedule depending on initial blood pressure. Results are for 40-year-old males and females under the age-varying partial benefit assumption. Under stepped control, treatment of diastolic blood pressures of 120 mm Hg is between two and three times as cost-effective as treatment of blood pressures of 100 mm Hg, with cost-effectiveness ranging from $3,200 and $3,900 per year saved for initial pressures of 120 mm Hg to $9,200 and $9,900 per year saved at 100 mm Hg for men and women respectively. The difference is even greater if it is assumed that control to 90 mm Hg is achieved.

The relationship between the cost-effectiveness ratio and the

---

5. As an extreme example, compare a man whose mortality rate each year is 0.9, lowered to 0.8, with a man whose mortality rate each year is 0.09, lowered to 0.08. The first man's life expectancy is increased from 1.11 years to 1.25 years, a gain of 0.14 years, while the second man's life expectancy is increased from 11.1 years to 12.5 years, a gain of 1.4 years.

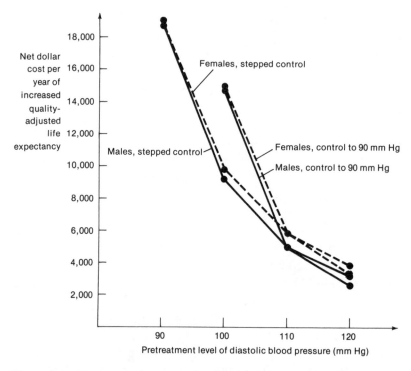

Figure 2.8: Effect of pretreatment blood pressure on cost-effectiveness of treatment. Results are given for the stepped control assumption and control to 90 mm Hg, for 40-year-old males and females. Assumes: age-varying partial benefit; discounting at 5 percent per annum; complete adherence to medical regimens.

diastolic blood pressure achieved by treatment for a 40-year-old with pretreatment diastolic pressures of 120, 110, and 100 mm Hg is shown in figure 2.9. The cost per year of life saved falls progressively as blood pressure is lowered. Most of the efficiency gains, however, are realized from the initial 10 mm Hg decrements, as indicated by the steeper slopes.

Figure 2.10 plots these same data in such a way as to indicate, for each pretreatment level, what controlled level must be achieved to justify treatment if $10,000 is determined to be the maximum allowable cost per year of quality-adjusted life saved. Note that the decrement of blood pressure required to achieve a given degree of efficiency (that is, to remain on the same iso-efficiency curve) becomes larger the lower the initial blood pressure. In males, for example, a decrement of 5 mm Hg from a pretreatment blood pressure of 120 mm Hg (from 120 mm Hg

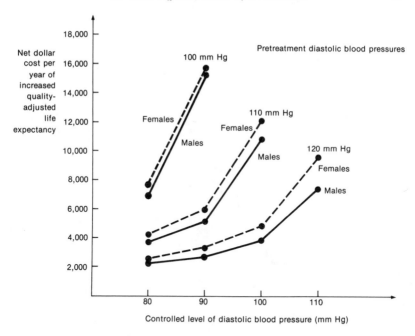

Figure 2.9: Cost-effectiveness for varying pretreatment and controlled blood pressures. Results apply to 40-year-old males and females. Assumes: age-varying partial benefit; discounting at 5 percent per annum; complete adherence to medical regimens.

to 115 mm Hg) is equivalent to a decrement of 12 mm Hg from a pretreatment blood pressure of 110 mm Hg.

RELATIONSHIPS AMONG COST-EFFECTIVENESS, AGE, AND PRETREATMENT BLOOD PRESSURE

The joint relationships among cost-effectiveness, age, and initial diastolic blood pressure are shown in figures 2.11 and 2.12 for males and females, respectively. For both sexes the cost-effectiveness ratio varies inversely with initial diastolic blood pressure. For males the ratio increases (equivalent to reduced cost-effectiveness) with age, while for females it decreases.

RELATIONSHIP OF COST-EFFECTIVENESS OF TREATMENT TO OTHER PATIENT CHARACTERISTICS

Other risk factors, including smoking habits, serum cholesterol, body weight, or the presence of diabetes mellitus, might be expected to influence the cost-effectiveness of antihypertensive treatment. For example, if smoking habits and hypertension are

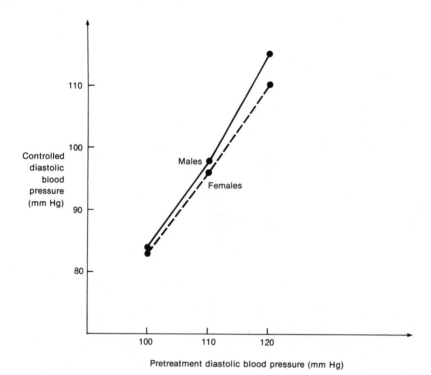

Pretreatment diastolic blood pressure (mm Hg)

Figure 2.10: Iso-efficiency curves by pretreatment and controlled levels of diastolic blood pressure. These are based upon a hypothetical maximum valuation of $10,000 per added quality-adjusted year of life expectancy, and are given for 40-year-old persons, by sex and pretreatment blood pressure. Assumes: age-varying partial benefit; discounting at 5 percent per annum, complete adherence to medical regimens.

multiplicative in their effects on mortality, a greater absolute reduction in mortality would be expected for hypertensive smokers than for hypertensive nonsmokers. Because life expectancy is shorter for smokers, however, the differences between the benefits of treatment for smokers and nonsmokers are not as great as might be expected.[6] For other risk factors, it is also possible that interactive effects enhance or diminish the effectiveness of antihypertensive treatment. Such possibilities were not evaluated, however.

6. For a 50-year-old male whose blood pressure is lowered from 110 mm Hg to 90 mm Hg, under the full benefit assumption, the increase in life expectancy has been computed to be 2.65 years for a smoker and 2.38 years for a nonsmoker [Shepard and Zeckhauser, 1974].

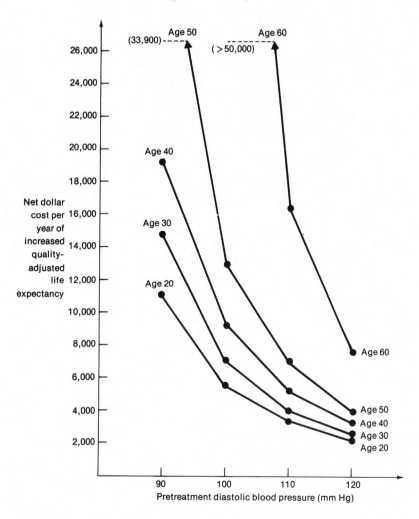

Figure 2.11: Cost-effectiveness for males by age and pretreatment level of diastolic blood pressure. Assumes: age-varying partial benefit; discounting at 5 percent per annum; stepped control; complete adherence to medical regimens.

The effect of the patient's medical condition on decisions to treat or not to treat was not explicitly considered in this analysis. Patients were assumed to be without evidence of coronary artery or cerebrovascular disease at the time treatment was begun. Because the relationship between decisions to treat blood pressure and associated clinical status of the patient has not been explicitly considered, and since treatment decisions and goals of treatment are frequently affected by the existence of such conditions as

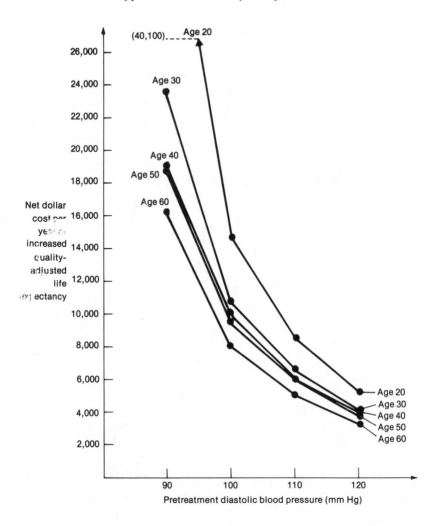

Figure 2.12: Cost-effectiveness for females by age and pretreatment level of diastolic blood pressure. Assumes: age-varying partial benefit; discounting at 5 percent per annum; stepped control; complete adherence to medical regimens.

angina pectoris or congestive heart failure, cost-effectiveness determinations would undoubtedly be altered in their presence. In the presence of congestive heart failure, for example, the cost-effectiveness of treatment will be greatly enhanced, at least in the short term, because the beneficial effect on cardiac function favorably affects both symptoms and prognosis.

IMPLICATIONS OF THE ANALYSIS FOR RESOURCE ALLOCATION

If treatment of high blood pressure paid for itself in the sense that the savings in later treatment of cardiovascular disease equalled or exceeded treatment costs, then the problem of resource allocation would not exist. Our findings indicate, however, that such is not the case. It is estimated that on average only 22 percent of gross treatment costs can be recovered from savings in the treatment of strokes and heart attacks in the United States adult population.[7] Under these conditions, the judgment of whether treatment is worthwhile rests upon the value attached to benefits received in the form of reduced mortality and morbidity, and it becomes essential to allocate resources to achieve the maximum possible benefit.

Decisions to allocate resources within hypertension or to alternative health care uses can reasonably be based on net cost per unit effectiveness conferred by treatment. From this analysis it is estimated that, if all United States adults with diastolic blood pressures of 105 mm Hg or above were treated, the aggregate cost-effectiveness would be $4,850 per year of increased quality-adjusted life expectancy. Treatment of "mild" hypertension between 95 mm Hg and 105 mm Hg would, however, cost $9,880 per year of increased quality-adjusted life expectancy.

Moreover, the analysis permits the selection of cutoff levels by pretreatment blood pressures, age, and sex for any chosen valuation of an added year of quality-adjusted life (figures 2.13 and 2.14). For any specified cost-effectiveness criterion, blood pressures above the corresponding curve should be treated. Thus, for example, if resource constraints dictate that the maximum permissible cost per year of life saved should be $10,000, the cutoff level for men aged 60 would be 117 mm Hg and for men aged 20 would be 92 mm Hg. For women the cutoff level falls with age from 107 mm Hg at age 20 to 97 mm Hg at age 60. For males, the blood pressure cutoff level rises with age because of the nature of the age-varying partial benefit assumption and because cardiovascular mortal and morbid events occur relatively early in life. Conversely, cutoff levels fall with age for females, though less markedly than the increase for males.

---

7. Based on treating all persons with diastolic blood pressures of 105 mm Hg and above.

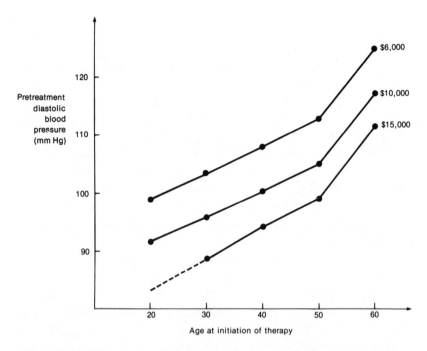

Figure 2.13: Criteria for treatment based on cost-effectiveness for males.
For any chosen valuation of an added year of quality-adjusted life, treatment should be provided for all age–blood pressure combinations *above*
the corresponding curve. Assumes: age-varying partial benefit; discounting at 5 percent per annum; stepped control; complete adherence to
medical regimens.

Cutoff levels of blood pressure determined by these cost-
effectiveness considerations are, in some instances, at odds with
commonly used clinical cutoff levels. Differences between the
objectives of involved decision makers and those that derive from
society's problem of resource allocation may, in part, be responsible.

Evaluation of the validity of these conclusions requires additional information, especially with regard to the effectiveness of
treatment and the incidence and impact on quality of life of
medication side effects. Even in their current form, however, they
do provide insights that can help decision makers with fixed
budgets, such has health maintenance organizations and community treatment programs, decide how to allocate their resources
to achieve maximum health benefits by the treatment of hypertension. As better information becomes available, these decisions
can be refined.

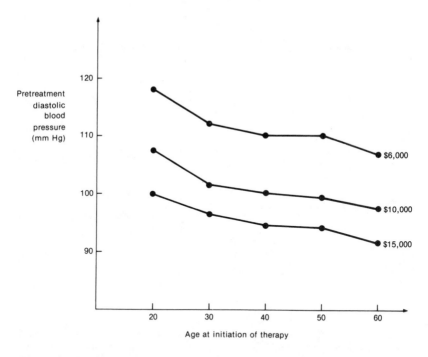

Figure 2.14: Criteria for treatment based on cost-effectiveness for females.
For any chosen valuation of an added year of quality-adjusted life, treatment should be provided for all age–blood pressure combinations *above*
the corresponding curve. Assumes: age-varying partial benefit; discounting at 5 percent per annum; stepped control; complete adherence to
medical regimens.

Furthermore, it should be emphasized that the analysis to
this point has assumed complete adherence to prescribed regimens. It is obvious that incomplete adherence will either decrease
the ability of prescribed therapy to achieve the assumed degrees
of blood pressure control, increase the cost of therapy as additional medications are prescribed in efforts to reach blood pressure goals, or both (see chapter 4). In any event the result is
a diminution in the cost-effectiveness of therapy. Results, therefore, represent upper bounds on cost-effectiveness or, alternatively, lower bounds of the cost per quality-adjusted life year
gained.

SENSITIVITY ANALYSIS

Assessment of the effects of variations in key parameters and
assumptions is a critical part of any analysis based on data that

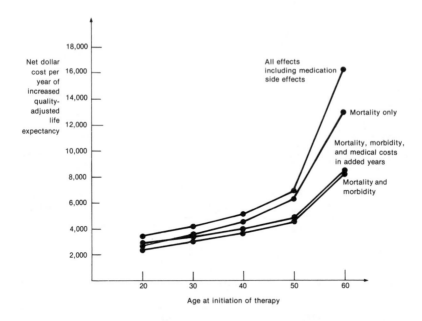

Figure 2.15: Impact on cost-effectiveness of morbidity benefits, medical costs in added years, and medication side effects, for males. Results by age at initiation of treatment are for a reduction in diastolic blood pressure from 110 mm Hg to 90 mm Hg. Assumes: age-varying partial benefit; discounting at 5 percent per annum; complete adherence to medical regimens.

are less than perfect. Conclusions that are not critically sensitive to variations in such parameters can be viewed with greater confidence; where extreme sensitivity is found, new information is needed.

EXPANSION OF THE ANALYSIS TO INCLUDE ALL COST AND EFFECTIVENESS PARAMETERS. Figures 2.15 and 2.16 expand the cost-effectiveness analysis stepwise from inclusion of mortality and treatment costs alone to inclusion, first, of the effects of reduced cardiovascular morbidity, second, of medical care costs in the added years of life expectancy, and, finally, of medication side effects. Cost-effectiveness is plotted against age at initiation of treatment for reductions in diastolic blood pressures from 110 mm Hg to 90 mm Hg under the age-varying partial benefit assumption. Comparative effects of each additional parameter are as follows:

• Side effects outweigh the benefits of reduced morbidity, except for older women, with resultant higher net costs per

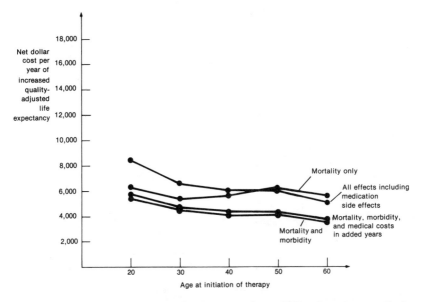

Figure 2.16: Impact on cost-effectiveness of morbidity benefits, medical costs in added years, and medication side effects, for females. Results by age at initiation of treatment are for a reduction in diastolic blood pressure from 110 mm Hg to 90 mm Hg. Assumes: age-varying partial benefit; discounting at 5 percent per annum; complete adherence to medical regimens.

quality-adjusted life year saved than when only mortality is included. The cost-effectiveness ratio remains under $10,000 for all groups except 60-year-old males;

• The relative importance of reduction in cardiovascular morbidity is greater in older age groups, despite the effect of the age-varying partial benefit assumption to favor treatment of the young; and

• The effect of the correction for medical costs associated with the treatment of noncardiovascular diseases that occur in the extended years of life is small.

The full data upon which figures 2.15 and 2.16 are based are given in tables 2A.4 and 2A.5 in the appendix to this chapter.

MEDICAL TREATMENT COSTS. Figure 2.17 displays the effect of several levels of antihypertensive treatment costs on the cost-effectiveness ratio. The average cost used throughout the analysis is $200. The lower and upper bounds examined here are $100 and $300, respectively. The cost per year of life saved is roughly proportional to changes in medical treatment costs. If drug costs

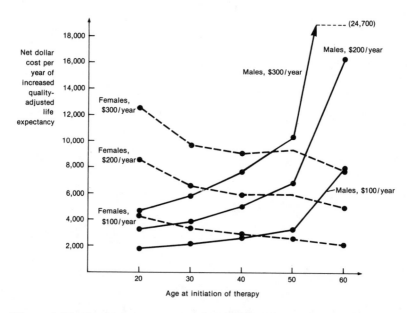

Figure 2.17: Sensitivity analysis, varying annual cost of antihypertensive treatment. Results are given for a range of annual treatment costs for a reduction in diastolic blood pressure from 110 mm Hg to 90 mm Hg. Assumes: age-varying partial benefit; discounting at 5 percent per annum; complete adherence to medical regimens.

represent about 70 percent of treatment costs, then a halving of drug costs would improve cost-effectiveness by more than one-third.

MEDICATION SIDE EFFECTS. The foregoing analysis assumed that the impairment in quality of life due to side effects from antihypertensive medications was such that an average patient would be willing to give up 1 percent of his life (1 year in 100 years or approximately 4 days in a year) to avoid them. Figure 2.18 shows the results of a sensitivity analysis in which side effects were assumed to be valued at 2 percent of one's total life years. This difference might reflect the varying frequency and severity of subjective side effects of different drugs (see chapter 3). The effects of this change are significant, especially in younger women and older men. If side effects are valued at 5 percent of total life years, the denominator of the cost-effectiveness ratio (that is, net effectiveness) actually becomes negative.

MEDICAL COSTS OF MORBID EVENTS AND VALUATION OF ALTERED QUALITY OF LIFE. The effects of variations in the costs of medical care for morbid events, and in the valuation of loss in

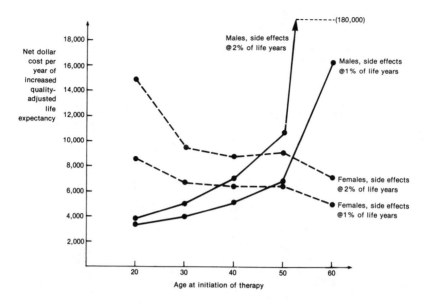

Figure 2.18: Sensitivity analysis, varying loss of quality of life due to treatment side effects. The imputed loss of either 1 percent or 2 percent of life years due to decreased quality of life from treatment side effects is examined. Results are for a reduction in diastolic blood pressure from 110 mm Hg to 90 mm Hg. Assumes: age-varying partial benefit; discounting at 5 percent per annum; complete adherence to medical regimens.

quality of life associated with myocardial infarctions and cerebro-vascular accidents, were examined. The assumption of $10,000 and 1.5 years per stroke and $7,000 and 0.5 years per myo-cardial infarction was contrasted with a "low" assumption of $7,000 and 1.0 years per stroke and $5,000 and 0.4 years per myocardial infarction, and with a "high" assumption of $15,000 and 2.0 years per stroke and $10,000 and 1.0 years per myo-cardial infarction. Because of the relatively small effect of morbidity on the cost-effectiveness ratio, the sensitivity to varia-tion in these assumptions is modest, as shown in figure 2.19. The analysis was less sensitive to these factors because their costs and values relative to the cost of antihypertensive treatment and the value of a year of life are small.

DISCOUNT RATE. The effect of the discount rate, noted pre-viously, is to alter the relative valuation of near-term and long-term costs and benefits. The higher the discount rate, the less the value attributed to savings of life years and improved quality of life in the future relative to costs and medication side effects

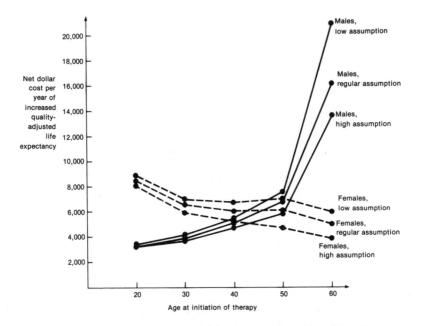

Figure 2.19: Sensitivity analysis comparing various assumptions regarding costs of morbid events. Low assumption is $7,000 and 1.0 life-year equivalents lost per stroke and $5,000 and 0.4 life-year equivalents lost per MI. Regular assumption is $10,000 and 1.5 life-year equivalents lost per stroke and $7,000 and 0.5 life-year equivalents lost per MI. High assumption is $15,000 and 2.0 life-year equivalents lost per stroke and $10,000 and 1.0 life-year equivalents lost per MI. Results are for a reduction in diastolic blood pressure from 110 mm Hg to 90 mm Hg. Assumes: age-varying partial benefit; discounting at 5 percent per annum; complete adherence to medical regimens.

in the present. The discount rate of 5 percent per annum used in the main analysis is contrasted here with discount rates of 0 percent (a lower bound reflecting no adjustment in benefits and costs for time) and 10 percent (an upper bound on discount rates used in policy analyses). As expected, the cost-effectiveness is rather sensitive to the choice of discount rate within these broad bounds (figure 2.20).

Policy Implications

This analysis, given its assumptions and the imperfect nature of information upon which it is based, indicates that greater cost-effectiveness is achieved by treating individuals with higher blood pressures, by initiating treatment at earlier ages in males than

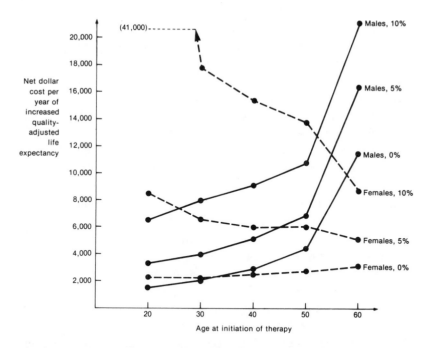

Figure 2.20: Sensitivity analysis with respect to discount rate. Cost-effectiveness of treatment is shown for discount rates of 0 percent (no discounting), 5 percent, and 10 percent. Results are for a reduction in diastolic blood pressure from 110 mm Hg to 90 mm Hg. Assumes: age-varying partial benefit; complete adherence to medical regimens.

females, and by attempting to control pressures to as low a level as possible consistent with tolerable side effects. These results permit setting priorities for treatment efforts based upon cost-effectiveness considerations (figures 2.13 and 2.14) rather than upon arbitrary criteria such as the number of standard deviations blood pressure is above the mean for age and sex.

NATIONAL RESOURCE IMPLICATIONS OF TREATING HYPER-TENSION

The annual national cost of treating all persons in the United States with diastolic blood pressures of 105 mm Hg and above is estimated at $1.4 billion.[8] If those "mild hypertensives" with diastolic pressures between 95 mm Hg and 105 mm Hg were also

8. This estimate and those that follow are based on the estimated 1975 United States adult population [Social Security Administration, 1974b], sex- and age-specific prevalences of hypertension [National Center for Health Statistics, 1964a], and an estimated annual treatment cost of $200.

treated, this annual cost would rise to $3.1 billion. Treatment of "borderline hypertensives" with diastolic pressures between 90 mm Hg and 95 mm Hg would further increase the annual cost to $4.8 billion. Clearly, the resource implications of treating mild and borderline hypertension are significant.

Unfortunately, it is highly unlikely that treatment of high blood pressure would pay for itself by reducing medical expenses for the treatment of cardiovascular disease. Because it is estimated that, on average, only 22 percent of antihypertensive treatment costs would be recovered from savings in the treatment of strokes and heart attacks in the United States adult population, the judgment of whether treatment is worthwhile must depend on the value attached to benefits received in the form of reduced mortality and improved quality of life.

Determination of the range of net dollar costs per year of life saved offers insight into the broader question of alternative use of scarce resources. Most would agree that if the cost per year of life saved were less than $1,000, major new resources should be allocated to hypertension programs. First, there are few areas of health care where treatment is so cost-effective and, second, there would be little disagreement that society should be willing to pay this much for a year of productive life. On the other hand, if the cost per year of life saved were in the millions of dollars, more efficient uses of resources could almost certainly be found. Cost-effectiveness ratios for hypertension treatment, however, fall within the range between $1,000 and $50,000 per year of life saved, a range that includes the annual earnings of most people, and, according to Acton [1973], the range that includes most people's willingness to pay to save a year of their own life. Aggregate national cost-effectiveness is estimated at $4,850 for treatment of moderate and severe hypertension (diastolic blood pressures of 105 mm Hg and above), and $9,880 for treatment of mild hypertension (diastolic blood pressures of 95 to 105 mm Hg). Widespread treatment of hypertension therefore appears to be neither an incredible bargain nor an extravagant misuse of scarce resources.

Mild hypertension is a special dilemma because of the uncertainty that surrounds both the clinical efficacy and cost-effectiveness of its treatment. Because it affects over 15 percent of the adult United States population (70 to 80 percent of "hypertensives" have diastolic blood pressures between 90 mm Hg and 105 mm Hg), it also poses major public policy questions. Currently it is not known with certainty whether treatment of blood pressure elevations in this range significantly diminishes cardiovascular risk. Moreover, cost-effectiveness estimates are extremely sensitive to the fraction of benefit achieved and the detrimental impact of drug side effects. Even if treatment is effective, more cost-effective uses of scarce resources might exist.

RESEARCH NEEDS

Additional information is needed to assess the fraction of benefit concept, especially for mild hypertension, and to quantify the degree and severity of medication side effects. The Hypertension Detection and Follow-up Program, a multicenter national program currently in progress, has as a major objective the ascertainment of benefit, particularly in mild hypertensives. Given a sufficient period of follow-up, it is hoped that useful data can be obtained.

To be realistic, however, it must be recognized that even the most carefully designed controlled studies rarely provide all the desired answers. Given this fact of life, resource allocation decisions cannot "wait until the final answers are in" before considering cost-effectiveness and will have to be made under conditions of uncertainty. It should be stressed in this regard that the conclusion should *not* be drawn from the Veterans Administration Study that treatment is *in*effective in preventing myocardial infarctions or in treating mild hypertension between 90 mm and 105 mm Hg diastolic. Reported results favor the treatment group by a small margin but were statistically insignificant. More extensive experience is needed before statistically valid conclusions can be drawn in either direction. Meanwhile, decisions continue to be made for such patients.

Information is urgently needed to assess the incidence, perceived severity, and costs of side effects of antihypertensive medications. The Boston Collaborative Drug Study has contributed greatly to our knowledge of adverse drug effects in hospitalized populations, but information on ambulatory hypertensive populations is sparse. Future investigations need to attempt to measure not only the incidence and characteristics of side effects but also the patient's perception of the degree of impact they have on the quality of life.

Another major area of research priority relates to treatment of younger individuals with elevated blood pressures. If the trend toward increased risk coefficients in younger age groups demonstrated in the Framingham Heart Study extends beyond the fourth decade to the third, second, or even first decade and, if the assumption of enhanced fraction of benefit in the young is true, then early detection and treatment in these groups will prove extremely cost-effective.

Appendix to Chapter 2

This appendix provides a more rigorous exposition of the methodology described in the text. Figure 2.3 gives an overview of the steps involved in the analysis. Each step will be discussed in turn, except where the discussion in the text is sufficiently detailed. The ultimate product is the calculation of the cost-effectiveness ratio,

$$\frac{C}{E} = \frac{\Delta C_{Rx} - \Delta C_{Morb} + \Delta C_{SE} + \Delta C_{Rx\triangle LE}}{\Delta Y_{LE} + \Delta Y_{Morb} - \Delta Y_{SE}}, \qquad (2A.1)$$

for each category of patient by sex, age, pretreatment and post-treatment blood pressure level (see text for categories of patients analyzed).

ESTIMATION OF AGE-SPECIFIC MORTALITY RATES. In the Framingham Heart Study [Kannel and Gordon, 1970, 1974] the relationship between diastolic blood pressure and two-year mortality for each decade between ages 35 and 74 and for both sexes has been fitted to the logistic risk function

$$q = 1/[1 + \exp(A - B \cdot BP)], \qquad (2A.2)$$

where q is two-year mortality, BP is diastolic blood pressure, B is a coefficient describing the contribution of blood pressure as a risk factor for each age and sex cohort, and A is a base risk or scaling factor for overall mortality in each age and sex cohort. Annual mortality was computed as $q/2$, a reasonable approximation of the exact formula $\sqrt{(1 + q)} - 1$ when q is small.

The A coefficients, or base risk coefficients, in the logistic risk function for mortality were corrected to account for the fact that the population selected for the Framingham Heart Study was healthier than the general population, being composed largely of individuals with no prior cardiovascular abnormalities.[1] This was done by estimating them for each decade and sex in such a

63

manner that the mortality rate computed from the risk function
($q/2$ in equation 2A.2) at the mean blood pressure for that
decade corresponds to the life table mortality rate for the mean
age of the decade.[2] The actual formula used to estimate A for
each decade is $A = B \cdot \overline{BP} + \ln[(.5/q_{\overline{BP}}) - 1]$, where $\overline{BP}$ is
the mean blood pressure at the mean age in the decade, and $q_{\overline{BP}}$
is the corresponding mortality rate from the life tables. This
was obtained by replacing q by $q/2$ in equation 2A.2, to convert
to annual mortality, and solving for A at the mean age and
blood pressure for the decade.

To examine the potential benefits of blood pressure control in
age groups younger than were included in the Framingham Heart
Study, the B coefficients of the risk function for the decade 35–44
were applied to the decades 15–24 and 25–34. Since the trend
is toward increasing coefficients at younger ages (see figure 2A.1),
this extrapolation is conservative in terms of estimating the benefits of blood pressure reduction in these age groups. Similar
extrapolations were used to estimate the B coefficients beyond age
74. Figure 2A.1 displays the B coefficients utilized in the analysis.
The A coefficients for the age groups outside the 35–74 range
were estimated independently by the procedure described above.

In using the Framingham risk data it was assumed that the
effect of the few individuals in the sample who were under treatment for hypertension was negligible. This assumption seems
justified by the fact that antihypertensive treatment for mild or
moderate asymptomatic hypertension was not standard medical
practice during most of the 18 years of the Framingham Study
prior to 1970. Hence, it is probable that very few patients were
under effective treatment. This is supported by the accelerating
rate of increase in blood pressure with age in the Framingham

---

1. The mortality of 40-year-old Framingham Study males with diastolic blood
pressure 90 mm Hg is lower than the mortality of New England white males
of the same age group with diastolic blood pressure of only 80 mm Hg.
2. The mean blood pressure for each decade was inferred from National
Health Examination Survey Data [National Center for Health Statistics,
1964a]. The mean age of a decade (for example, 35–44) was calculated as
the statistical mean of the distribution of ages within the decade, based on
the life tables [National Center for Health Statistics, 1968]. The mortality rate
at the mean blood pressure of a decade is somewhat of an overestimate of
the mean mortality rate for the decade because of the convexity of the risk
curve as a function of blood pressure (figure 2.1), but the error introduced
was found to be negligible.

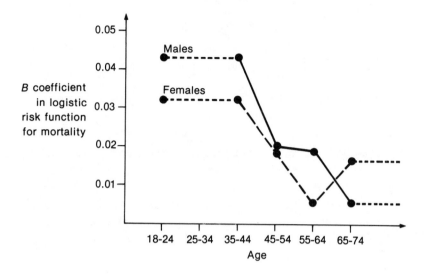

Figure 2A.1: Mortality risk coefficient (B) extrapolations. B coefficients in the risk function

$$q = 1/2[1 + \exp(A - B \cdot BP)]^{-1}$$

for the decade 35–44 were extended to apply to ages 18–34 and that for the decade 65–74 to ages greater than 74. (Source: Framingham Heart Study [Kannel and Gordon, 1970, 1974].)

cohort [Feinleib, 1974], an effect that would not have been as pronounced if a significant and increasing number of individuals were having their blood pressures lowered during the course of the study.

RISE OF BLOOD PRESSURE WITH AGE. The change of blood pressure with age was estimated under two assumptions, referred to as the "unadjusted" and the "adjusted" natural history assumptions. The "unadjusted" assumption holds that the absolute increment in blood pressure with each decade is the same as the mean change obtained from the cross-sectional National Health Examination Survey [National Center for Health Statistics, 1964a]. The "adjusted" assumption, on the other hand, recognizes that cross-sectional data on mean blood pressure tend to underestimate the rate of increase with age because of the selective survival of individuals with low blood pressures, and it adjusts for this bias by assuming that blood pressure continues to rise with age at the slope found to hold during the decade just prior to the leveling off. Except where otherwise noted, the adjusted natural history assumption was employed throughout, though sensitivity analysis indicated almost no difference between the two.

For patients under blood pressure control, it was assumed that only a fraction of the natural rise occurs. This fraction of control parameter was set at 0.5 for the present analysis. Thus, if the uncontrolled diastolic blood pressure would rise by Δx mm Hg during a given age decade (as computed by the adjusted natural history assumption), then the controlled diastolic blood pressure was assumed to rise by $0.5\Delta x$ mm Hg during that decade. The updating of blood pressure was done once each decade (at year $10n + 5$), and blood pressure was assumed constant throughout the decade.

CALCULATION OF LIFE EXPECTANCY FOR UNCONTROLLED BLOOD PRESSURES.   Survival curves were generated for men and women, ages 20, 30, 40, 50, and 60, with uncontrolled diastolic blood pressures ranging from 90 mm Hg to 120 mm Hg. This was done by (1) computing from the logistic risk function (equation 2A.1), with parameters as described above, the annual mortality rate by sex, initial age, and pretreatment blood pressure; (2) taking the ratio of this mortality rate to the life table mortality rate for the mean age in that decade; (3) multiplying the age-specific life table mortalities by this ratio to derive mortality rates for each of the remaining five years in the initial decade (for example, 40–44 for initial age 40); (4) calculating the subject's expected blood pressure in the next decade under the adjusted natural history assumption; (5) computing from the risk function the annual mortality rate for the next full decade at the updated blood pressure level; (6) taking the ratio of this mortality rate to the life table mortality rate for the mean age in that next decade; (7) multiplying the age-specific life table mortalities by this ratio to derive mortality rates for each year in the next decade (for example, 45–54 for initial age 40); (8) repeating steps (4) through (7) up to age 74; (9) continuing beyond age 74 without updating blood pressure and using the risk ratio corresponding to the decade 65–74.

Life expectancy for each age–sex–blood pressure group was then computed from the derived schedule of mortality rates by the usual method of summing cumulative annual survival rates. Specifically, if M_i is the computed mortality rate from age i to age $i + 1$ for an individual who is currently at age i_0, then the survival rate to age j is given by

$$S_j = \prod_{i=i_0}^{j-1} (1 - M_i),$$

and remaining life expectancy is given by

$$LE = \sum_{j=i_0}^{\infty} S_i.$$

Discounted remaining life expectancy, which counts year $i_0 + t$ as only $(1 + r)^{-t}$ as much as year i_0, is given by

$$LE_{Disc} = \sum_{j=i_0}^{\infty} S_i (1 + r)^{-t}.$$

The value of $r = 0.05$ was used in the analysis.

CALCULATION OF LIFE EXPECTANCY FOR CONTROLLED BLOOD PRESSURES. Each age-specific mortality rate for patients under blood pressure control was estimated as a weighted average of the mortality rate corresponding to the actual blood pressure and that corresponding to the blood pressure level that would have occurred in the absence of control. The weight is the fraction of benefit (FOB). Thus if m_i is the mortality at the lower (controlled) level, and M_i is the mortality at the higher (uncontrolled) level, then the computed mortality is given by

$$\overline{m} = m_i f_{(i,\ i-i_0)} + M_i (1 - f_{(i,\ i-i_0)}),$$

where $f_{(i_0,\ i-i_0)}$ is the FOB coefficient for a person who initiated treatment at age i_0 and whose blood pressure has been controlled for $i - i_0$ years (see table 2.1 for the parameters of the age-varying partial benefit assumption).

Given this schedule of mortality rates, $\overline{m}_i$, life expectancy ($\overline{LE}$) and discounted life expectancy ($\overline{LE_{Disc}}$) were computed as described for uncontrolled blood pressures. The increase in discounted life expectancy between the controlled and uncontrolled cases is the term ΔY_{LE} in the denominator of the cost-effectiveness ratio (equation 2A.1):

$$\Delta Y_{LE} = \overline{LE_{Disc}} - LE_{Disc}.$$

ESTIMATION OF THE COST OF A LIFETIME OF ANTIHYPERTEN-
SIVE TREATMENT.   The annual cost of treatment, c, was taken to
be $200. An additional first-year diagnostic cost of $100 was
added. Thus, the expected net present value lifetime cost of
treatment for each sex, age, pretreatment and posttreatment
blood pressure was estimated as

$$\Delta C_{Rx} = 100 + c \cdot \overline{LE}_{Disc},$$

where $\overline{LE}_{Disc}$ is life expectancy under control, and ΔC_{Rx} becomes
the first term in the numerator of the cost-effectiveness ratio
(equation 2A.1).

ESTIMATION OF MORBIDITY RATES AND EXPECTED LIFETIME
INCIDENCE OF STROKE AND MYOCARDIAL INFARCTION.   Events
were defined as in the Framingham Heart Study and were limited
to first events of each kind. The method for handling recurrences
is discussed subsequently. Incidence rates for stroke (CVA) and
myocardial infarction (MI) by age, sex, and uncontrolled blood
pressure were taken from the Framingham data and applied in
each year of life to the proportion of the population surviving
and previously free of the event. As for mortality, B coefficients
were extrapolated to below age 35 and above age 74 by applying
the values for the decades 35–44 and 65–74 respectively. The
A coefficients were taken as given. Incidence curves for CVA and
MI were computed by the procedure used for mortality, except
that average age-specific Framingham incidence rates for CVA
and MI played the role of life-table mortality rates in the adjustment procedure. Incidence rates for individuals under blood
pressure control were then calculated under the alternative fraction of benefit assumptions (see table 2.2 for the parameters of
the age-varying partial benefit assumption) by the same method
as for mortality.

The expected lifetime incidence of CVA and MI was com-
puted as follows. Let p_i and $\bar{p}_i$ be the annual incidence probabilities, conditional upon survival to age i without an event, for the
uncontrolled and controlled patient, respectively. Let s_i and $\bar{s}_i$ be
the corresponding cumulative survival rates, and let d be the
fatality rate for the morbid event. Then the incidence of the event
in year j (q_j or $\bar{q}_j$) is given by the probability of surviving to year
j without an event, multiplied by the probability of a new event in
that year:

$$q_j = s_j \prod_{i=t_c}^{j-1} [1 - (1 - d)\bar{p}_i]$$

and

$$\bar{q}_j = \bar{s}_j \prod_{i=i_0}^{j-1} [1 - (1 - d)\bar{p}_i].$$

The decrease in expected lifetime incidence (ΔQ) is then given by

$$\Delta Q = \sum_{j=i_0}^{\infty} (q_j - \bar{q}_j).$$

In addition to the net change in the expected lifetime incidence of strokes (CVA) and myocardial infarctions (MI), the net change in the *discounted* expected lifetime incidence of CVA and MI was also computed. For example, a CVA occurring ten years after initiation of therapy counted as $1/1.05^{10}$ of a present-value CVA in the computation of the expected number of events. The decrease in discounted expected lifetime incidence (ΔQ_{Disc}) was computed as

$$\Delta Q_{Disc} = \sum_{j=i_0}^{\infty} (q_j - \bar{q}_j)(1 + r)^{j-i_0}.$$

VALUATION OF IMPROVEMENT IN QUALITY OF LIFE FROM REDUCED CARDIOVASCULAR MORBIDITY. For stroke, results of a study by Emlet et al. [1973] were used to provide estimates of disability. In that study, a panel of experts assessed, for each of four classes of stroke victims, the expected number of years spent in each of five disability states following a first stroke, including the effects of recurrent strokes. These are shown in table 2A.1, together with our own estimates for the remaining nonfatal stroke victims who are mildly affected and for those who die. The top row of table 2A.1 gives a subjective valuation of the life-year equivalent cost per year in each disability state.

The equivalent number of life years lost per incident stroke for each patient category was computed as follows. First, each expected year of disability was discounted back to the time of the incident stroke at 5 percent per year, assuming that the most severe disability occurred first. (This assumption is more valid for patients who recover than for those who get progressively worse and then die, but fortunately the results are not at all sensitive to this assumption.) Next, the numbers of present-value years in each state were multiplied by the corresponding life-year equivalent cost, and summed, to give the expected discounted number of life-year equivalents lost per incident stroke. These results are found in the next to last column of table 2A.1.

Table 2A.1: Calculation of life-year equivalent loss associated with morbid effects of an initial stroke.

Patient group[a]	Disability states					Equivalent life years lost (present value at 5% per annum)	Frequency of cases
	Totally dependent	Partially dependent	Requiring supervision	Capable of self care	Detectable/ symptomatic		
Equivalent life years lost per year in disability state	0.9	0.8	0.5	0.2	0.05		
Years spent in disability state							
A	1.6	0.5	0.2	0	0	1.9	0.077
B	0.8	2.0	1.4	0.8	0	3.2	.152
C	0.3	1.6	4.0	4.8	4.4	4.7	.100
D	0.4	1.3	2.1	1.5	0.6	2.8	.105
Other nonfatal	0	0.1	0	1.0	0	0.3	.366
Deaths	0	0	0	0	0	0	.200
Weighted average by frequency of cases	—	—	—	—	—	1.5 years	—

a Group A: ≥55 years, marked impairment; B: ≥55 years, moderate impairment; C: <55 years, mild impairment; D: ≥55 years, mild impairment [Emlet et al., 1973]. Data for other nonfatal cases and deaths are our judgmental estimates.

Finally, the expected life-year equivalents lost per incident stroke were averaged over all patient categories, using the frequencies shown in the last column of table 2A.1 (Emlet et al., 1973). This resulted in an estimate of 1.5 life-year equivalents lost per incident stroke due to morbidity and disability.

For myocardial infarction, exactly the same methods were used, although the data used were our own estimates, and the result was an estimate of 0.5 life-year equivalents lost per incident MI due to morbidity and disability (table 2A.2).

The procedure used automatically accounts for recurrent events, and automatically discounts morbid effects back to the time of the incident event. Discounting to the present (that is, the time of initiation of antihypertensive therapy) is accomplished by the use of the discounted expected lifetime incidence of morbid events as described above.

The change in quality of life is computed as

$$\Delta Y_{Morb} = \Delta Q_{Disc}^{CVA} \cdot 1.5 + \Delta Q_{Disc}^{MI} \cdot 0.5,$$

Table 2A.2: Calculation of life-year equivalent loss associated with morbid effects of an initial myocardial infarction.

Patient group	Disability states			Equivalent life-years lost (present value at 5% per annum)	Frequency of cases
	Requiring super-vision	Capable of self care	Detect-able/ sympto-matic		
	Equivalent life years lost per year in disability state				
	0.5	0.2	0.05		
	Years spent in disability state				
No residual disability	0.05	0	10	0.4	0.75
Disabled	0.05	10	0	2.0	.10
Dead	0	0	0	0	.15
Weighted average by frequency of cases	—	—	—	0.5 years	—

All data are our judgmental estimates. Definition of MI used was that of the Framingham Heart Study which effectively excludes sudden deaths. Mortality estimate is therefore for hospitalized patients.

and this term appears as an adjustment to life expectancy in the denominator of the cost-effectiveness ratio (equation 2A.1).

ESTIMATION OF COST SAVINGS FROM CARDIOVASCULAR MORBIDITY PREVENTED

The panel of experts in the study by Emlet et al. [1973] estimated the expected present-value lifetime medical costs subsequent to an initial stroke for each of four categories of stroke victims. These are shown in table 2A.3, along with our own subjective estimates for other nonfatal strokes and for fatal strokes. Costs per case were weighted by the frequencies of the patient categories to yield the average present-value cost per incident stroke. An inflation factor of 15 percent was incorporated to bring the estimates up to 1976 price levels.

For myocardial infarction, using the Framingham definition which excludes sudden deaths, the cost of care per event was estimated from Medicare data to be $3,000 [Social Security Administration, 1974b]. This represents a weighted average of $3,500 for a nonfatal MI and $500 for a fatal MI, assuming a hospital mortality rate of 17 percent. Using the estimated proba-

Table 2A.3: Calculation of cost per incident stroke. Estimate of $8,500 in 1972 is inflated at 15 percent per year to approximately $10,000 in 1976.

Patient group[a]	Frequency of cases	Lifetime cost per case in thousands of dollars
A	0.077	31.0
B	.152	17.1
C	.100	7.6
D	.105	8.0
Other nonfatal	.366	5.0
Deaths	.200	0.5
Weighted average by frequency of cases	—	8.5

[a] Group A: ≥ 55 years, marked impairment; B: ≥ 55 years, moderate impairment; C: < 55 years, mild impairment; D: ≥ 55 years, mild impairment [Emlet et al., 1973]. Data for other nonfatal cases and deaths are our judgmental estimates.

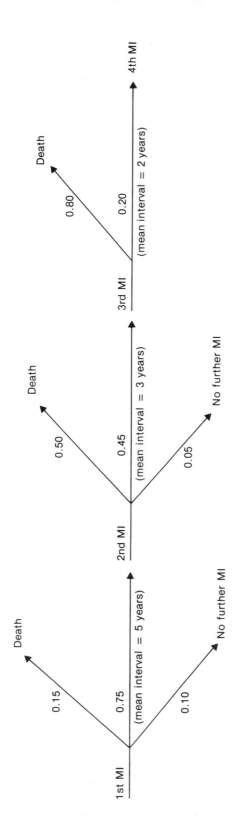

Figure 2A.2: Probabilities of recurrences of myocardial infarction and their outcomes. All probability estimates are judgmental. For the first MI the Framingham Heart Study definition is used, and hence the probability of death is only that for hospitalized patients. For all subsequent MIs the probability of death includes both sudden (out-of-hospital) and hospital deaths.

bilities of recurrence shown in figure 2A.2, the expected discounted hospital cost per case (not per MI) was computed:

$$\text{Cost per case} = \sum_{i=1}^{4} s_i[m_i C_D + (1 - m_i)C_S](1 + r)^{-t_i}$$

$$= [(.15)(500) + (.85)(3500)]$$

$$+ \frac{(.75)[(.5)(500) + (.5)(3500)]}{(1.05)^5}$$

$$+ \frac{(.75)(.45)[(.8)(500) + (.2)(3500)]}{(1.05)^8}$$

$$+ \frac{(.75)(.45)(.2)(500)}{(1.05)^{10}}$$

$$\cong \$4,500,$$

where:

s_i = probability of having at least i MIs, given the first;
m_i = probability of death from the ith MI;
C_D = cost of acute care for fatal MI (= \$500);
C_S = cost of acute care for nonfatal MI (= \$3,500);
r = discount rate (= 0.05);
t_i = expected time between first MI and ith MI;

and where possible hospitalizations for heart problems other than acute MI are not included. Expected present-value lifetime medical costs per case, excluding the cost of hospitalization for treatment of MI and possible coronary artery surgery, were estimated at about \$2,500 by assuming an annual average cost of \$160 for a lifetime of twenty years, discounted at 5 percent per year. Hence, an estimate of the total medical costs saved per initial MI prevented (discounted back to the time of the initial event) is \$7,000.

The cost savings are computed as

$$\Delta C_{Morb} = \Delta Q_{Disc}^{CVA} \cdot \$10,000 + \Delta Q_{Disc}^{MI} \cdot \$7,000,$$

and this term appears in the numerator of the cost-effectiveness ratio (equation 2A.1).

VALUATION OF IMPAIRMENT OF QUALITY OF LIFE DUE TO TREATMENT SIDE EFFECTS. The net influence on quality of life of the therapeutic regimen is assumed to be equivalent to an x percent reduction in the effective discounted life expectancy.

Thus, the term ΔY_{SE} in the denominator of the cost-effectiveness ratio (equation 2A.1) is defined by

$$\Delta Y_{SE} = (x/100)\overline{LE}_{Disc}.$$

In the main analysis x was taken to be 1, reflecting the equivalent

Table 2A.4: Cost-effectiveness data for males by age and pretreatment diastolic blood pressure.

Age	Initial diastolic blood pressure (mm Hg)	Controlled diastolic blood pressure (mm Hg)	Life expectancy, discounted	Discounted change in life expectancy	Adjustment to discounted change in life expectancy for cardiovascular morbidity (+)	Adjustment to discounted change in life expectancy for side effects (−)	Discounted lifetime treatment cost ($)	Discounted savings in medical costs for cardiovascular morbidity ($)	Discounted medical costs in added years ($)	Discounted costs of side effects ($)	Net cost per year of increased quality-adjusted life expectancy ($)
20	90	80	18.30	0.53	0.01	0.18	3760	94	159	125	10,970
	100	85	18.04	0.88	.02	.18	3708	134	264	125	5,500
	110	90	17.72	1.37	.03	.18	3644	194	411	125	3,270
	120	95	17.32	2.03	.04	.17	3564	257	609	125	2,130
30	90	80	17.12	0.41	.01	.17	3524	94	123	125	14,700
	100	85	16.80	0.67	.02	.17	3460	178	201	125	6,940
	110	90	16.39	1.00	.04	.16	3378	285	300	125	4,000
	120	95	15.87	1.43	.06	.16	3274	415	429	125	2,570
40	90	80	15.28	0.30	.02	.15	3156	114	90	125	19,150
	100	85	14.89	0.46	.03	.15	3078	201	138	125	9,230
	110	90	14.42	0.66	.05	.14	2984	348	198	125	5,190
	120	95	13.84	0.90	.08	.14	2686	565	270	125	3,210
50	90	80	12.77	0.19	.02	.13	2654	124	57	125	33,880
	100	85	12.39	0.29	.03	.12	2578	224	87	125	12,820
	110	90	11.98	0.40	.06	.12	2498	407	120	125	6,870
	120	95	11.53	0.51	.11	.12	2406	724	153	125	3,920
60	90	80	9.94	0.08	.01	.10	2088	87	24	125	Undefined
	100	85	9.61	0.11	.03	.10	2022	174	33	125	50,100
	110	90	9.26	0.15	.05	.09	1952	324	45	125	16,330
	120	95	8.88	0.19	.09	.09	1876	584	57	125	7,750

Assumes: age-varying partial benefit; discounting at 5% per annum; stepped control; complete adherence to medical regimens.

Table 2A.5: Cost-effectiveness data for females by age and pretreatment diastolic blood pressure.

Age	Initial diastolic blood pressure (mm Hg)	Controlled diastolic blood pressure (mm Hg)	Life expectancy, discounted	Discounted change in life expectancy	Adjustment to discounted change in life expectancy for cardiovascular morbidity (+)	Adjustment to discounted change in life expectancy for side effects (−)	Discounted lifetime treatment cost ($)	Discounted savings in medical costs for cardiovascular morbidity ($)	Discounted medical costs in added years ($)	Discounted costs of side effects ($)	Net cost per year of increased quality-adjusted life expectancy ($)
20	90	80	19.09	0.27	0.02	0.19	3918	114	81	125	40,080
	100	85	18.99	.43	.03	.19	3898	188	129	125	14,670
	110	90	18.87	.61	.04	.19	3874	275	183	125	8,490
	120	95	18.74	.86	.06	.19	3848	392	258	125	5,260
30	90	80	18.07	.32	.02	.18	3714	161	96	125	23,580
	100	85	17.92	.49	.04	.18	3684	255	147	125	10,570
	110	90	17.74	.68	.05	.18	3648	389	204	125	6,520
	120	95	17.55	.94	.08	.18	3610	573	282	125	4,100
40	90	80	16.55	.32	.03	.17	3410	218	96	125	18,950
	100	85	16.32	.44	.05	.16	3364	359	132	125	9,880
	110	90	16.08	.59	.08	.16	3316	560	177	125	5,990
	120	95	15.80	.75	.12	.16	3260	828	225	125	3,920
50	90	80	14.52	.28	.03	.15	3004	228	84	125	18,640
	100	85	14.28	.38	.06	.14	2956	406	114	125	9,290
	110	90	14.02	.47	.09	.14	2904	647	141	125	6,000
	120	95	13.75	.56	.14	.14	2850	989	168	125	3,840
60	90	80	11.80	.24	.03	.12	2460	221	72	125	16,230
	100	85	11.47	.33	.06	.11	2394	385	99	125	7,970
	110	90	11.13	.41	.09	.11	2326	609	123	125	5,030
	120	95	10.79	.48	.13	.11	2258	917	144	125	3,220

Assumes: age-varying partial benefit; discounting at 5% per annum; stepped control; complete adherence to medical regimens.

of a one percent reduction in effective life expectancy when under antihypertensive therapy.

ESTIMATION OF THE COSTS OF TREATING MEDICATION SIDE EFFECTS. It was assumed that $\Delta C_{SE} = \$125$ (present value) for all patients (see chapter 3).

ESTIMATION OF MEDICAL COSTS INCURRED IN THE ADDED YEARS OF LIFE EXPECTANCY. It was assumed that $\Delta C_{R_x \Delta LE} = \$300 \cdot \Delta Y_{LE}$ for all patients, reflecting an average annual expenditure of $300 on noncardiovascular medical care during the added years of life (see text). This is automatically converted to present value through the discounting embodied in the term ΔY_{LE}.

RESULTS. The detailed breakdown of cost-effectiveness results under the basic assumptions used, for each patient category by age and blood pressure, is given in table 2A.4 for males and table 2A.5 for females.

3. Drug Side Effects and the Cost-Effectiveness of Treatment

"The heavy dosage was not without its side effects. Sphincter control became a problem. There was frequency of bowel motions and an urgency of urination which affected my social life and work. As a doctor I doubt whether I could have asked a patient to endure such treatment . . . After six months my systolic pressure fell slowly from 200 to 140 mm Hg, but my diastolic pressure persisted at 120 . . . The methyldopa had been reinforced by chlorothiazide, and for many months I felt weakness and incompetence of thigh and shoulder muscles, which soon disappeared with an aperitif of orange juice. Then came an attack of gout—typically in the first instance in the right great toe, but spreading to all the toes—both left and right. Chlorothiazide was discarded and the newest diuretic substituted. Chlorthalidone was the favorite. The gout disappeared . . . Over the next twelve months my weight fell gradually from fourteen to eleven and a half stone. I had frequent attacks of tachycardia [rapid heart beat] when my pulse was uncountable and I merely felt a continuous flow. Suddenly I would be drenched with sweat, and I sat with a curious sense of angor animi [a feeling of impending dissolution]. My nights were disturbed with polyuria [excessive urination]. But it was my loss of weight that eventually took me to my physician. He found that I had a ketonuria of 4 plus and a glycosuria of 4 plus [symptoms of diabetes mellitus]. I eventually went to the hospital, stopped all pills, had my insulin standardized, and on my first blood sugar check a fortnight later

---

Note: The authors of this chapter are David Blumenthal, William B. Stason, and Milton C. Weinstein.

I came off all treatment [for diabetes]. That night the year book on endocrinology arrived, and I opened it at the series of articles describing the iatrogenic [treatment-induced] effect of chlorthalidone. All of this happened five years ago. The dose of methyldopa has gone down to two tablets a day. My blood sugar is normal, my blood urea is normal, and my blood pressure is 140/90. Obviously if you can survive the treatment there is hope at the other end" (from "History of a Hypertensive," *Lancet,* December 9, 1972).

The public is well aware that buying drugs can be expensive. As physicians well know, however, the cost of a drug purchase may not constitute the full cost of its ingestion. Few, if any, medications accomplish their therapeutic purposes without exacting some price in the form of unintended ill effects on the health and well-being of their consumers. Drug side effects add to the dollar cost of treating disease by creating ailments which themselves require medical treatment for amelioration or cure. They also diminish the quality of life for the patient and may, occasionally, lead to death.

Drug side effects are important considerations when embarking on any treatment regimen, regardless of the drug or disease at issue. They are of special concern in the treatment of essential hypertension, for several reasons. First, antihypertensive medications commonly in use today are known to induce distressing, crippling, or even fatal drug reactions. Second, treatment regimens often commit relatively young patients to a lifetime of drug use. Third, essential hypertension, especially in its mild variety, is widespread, affecting well over 20 million Americans [National High Blood Pressure Education Program, 1973e]. Fourth, governmental authorities and voluntary agencies have initiated broad-ranging efforts to encourage hypertensives to seek treatment for their disease [Stokes and Ward, 1974; *Time,* 1975].

These circumstances argue for giving careful consideration to the impact of the side effects of medications when assessing the cost-effectiveness of antihypertensive treatment. This chapter examines this question in a quantitative manner by focusing on (1) the incremental annual costs associated with the medical treatment of specific drug side effects; and (2) the increments in age-specific mortality rates attributable to the occurrence of fatal drug side effects.

Another parameter of equal or even greater importance is the diminution of quality of life associated with the mild, long-term effects of medication. Clearly the quality of ensuing life is a major outcome of any therapeutic intervention, and the valuation placed on other outcomes, including life years saved, is heavily influenced by the conditions under which such years are lived. In chapter 2 cost-effectiveness of treatment was, in fact, shown to be highly sensitive to the impact of subjective side effects on the quality of life. Because no data exist to assess these effects more rigorously than was done there, they will not be dealt with in detail in this chapter.

Available Treatment Regimens and Their Costs

A substantial array of drugs is currently available for lowering blood pressure, and new medications are continually being added to the physician's therapeutic armamentarium. At present, however, four basic regimens have gained wide popularity for the control of uncomplicated hypertension in ambulatory settings. These are:

diuretic only (usually a benzothiadiazide or thiazide),
diuretic + reserpine,
diuretic + alpha-methyldopa, and
diuretic + hydralazine + propranolol.

The first three of these are evaluated in this analysis.

A diuretic alone is frequently effective in controlling mild hypertension and, in any case, physicians usually initiate therapy with a diuretic and add additional medications as required. Figure 3.1 shows the drug protocol recommended by the National High Blood Pressure Education Program [1973b]. Note that the alternative regimens are recommended only for patients with diastolic blood pressures between 105 mm Hg and 140 mm Hg. Below such levels individualized treatment regimens are recommended.

Other than medication side effects, two important kinds of costs associated with long-term drug therapy for hypertension can be identified. The first of these is the monetary cost. Estimated annual treatment costs are presented in table 3.1. These reflect the fact that management of high blood pressure involves initial expenditures to evaluate patients for curable causes of hyperten-

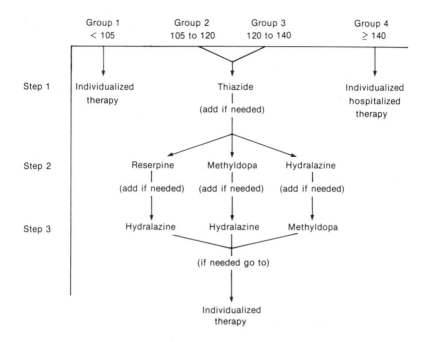

Figure 3.1: Outline of recommended antihypertensive regimens for groups with varyingly severe hypertension as indicated by diastolic blood pressure (mm Hg). The therapeutic objective of these regimens is to achieve a diastolic pressure under 90 mm Hg or, if untoward effects cannot be tolerated, under 100 mm Hg. (Source: National High Blood Pressure Education Program [1973b].)

sion.[1] For patients with essential hypertension, treatment increases the frequency with which the patient must visit his physician, and adds the costs of the medications themselves and of the laboratory examinations required to monitor for the possible development of side effects. The annual incremental cost of treating hypertension ranges from $157 to $411 depending on the drugs used. The patient can expect to pay this amount each year for the remainder of his or her life.

A second cost is the inconvenience involved in taking antihypertensive medications. Some patients find that drug-taking significantly interferes with their daily routines and is a source of great annoyance. Though this may seem a trivial matter in the abstract, it is sufficiently important to some patients

---

1. See chapter 7 for an analysis of the costs and benefits of such evaluations and subsequent treatment.

Table 3.1: Expected annual cost of treatment for mild and moderate essential hypertension.[a]

Expenses	Physicians' fees	Medi-cations	Lab work (routine)	Lab work (optional)	Total
First year					
Evaluation for curable causes of hypertension	$44	—	$71[b]	$120[c]	$235
Annual					
Diuretic only	54[d]	$ 83[e]	20[f]	—	157
Diuretic and reserpine	54	112[g]	20[f]	—	186
Diuretic and methyldopa	54	180[h]	27[i]	—	261
Diuretic, hydralazine, and propranolol	54	328[j]	29	—	411

[a] Costs of physician visits and laboratory services based on Massachusetts General Hospital prices, 1975. Drug prices calculated by doubling price to the retailer [*Drug Topics Red Book,* 1975].
[b] Includes serum creatinine, potassium, uric acid, cholesterol, blood sugar, hematocrit, chest x-ray, electrocardiogram, and urinalysis (without sediment).
[c] Includes intravenous pyelogram, urinary catecholamines, and two plasma renin determinations.
[d] Assumes the patient visits a physician three more times per year than if he were not hypertensive.
[e] Chlorothiazide 1,000 mg a day.
[f] Includes two serum potassium determinations, two uric acid determinations, two blood sugar determinations.
[g] Chlorothiazide, 1,000 mg a day; reserpine, 0.25 mg a day.
[h] Chlorothiazide, 1,000 mg a day; alpha-methyldopa, 500 mg a day.
[i] Same as note f above, plus a direct Coombs test yearly.
[j] Chlorothiazide, 1,000 mg a day; hydralazine, 100 mg a day; propranolol, 160 mg a day.

to result in their discontinuing therapy. Because antihypertensive therapy commits the patient to decades of daily drug ingestion, often involving multiple pills taken three to four times daily, the cost imposed may be considerable.[2]

Side Effects as Iatrogenic Diseases

The side effects of drugs can be viewed as treatment-induced, or iatrogenic, diseases. Like all diseases, they can occur in mild or severe forms and have variable durations, in many cases heavily influenced by whether or not drug administration is continued. They may carry risks of death or of morbidity sufficient to require ambulatory or even hospital treatment. In analyzing

2. In the analysis of chapter 2, inconvenience was treated as a subjective side effect of therapy.

the impact of these on the cost-effectiveness of treatment, attention must be directed at delineating the following characteristics of each iatrogenic disease:

• the incremental annual probability that the drug-taker will experience the disease when he is taking the drug as opposed to when he is not;
• the natural history of the disease;
• the probability that an individual with the stated disease will be hospitalized for treatment;
• the increment in age-specific death rates, if any, resulting from the development of the particular disease.

Taking the difference between the probability of experiencing a disease when a patient is taking the drug as opposed to when he is not accounts for the fact that many of the conditions identified as side effects also occur in individuals who are not taking the drug. Interest is in the extent to which drug ingestion adds to the probability that the condition will occur, rather than in its absolute incidence.

The natural history is important because it helps to predict the distribution over time of the consequences of the disease in question. In calculating the time stream of dollar costs associated with drug-induced disease, knowledge of the natural history permits application of the principles of discounting in valuing expenditures that are likely to occur well in the future. Further, it is a prerequisite to the estimation of the age-specific death rates and hence of life expectancy.

The probability that the disease will require hospitalization is important because hospital care will usually constitute a substantial proportion of any costs of treatment. Moreover, hospitalization entails limitation of activity and possibly some loss of earnings for the patient, although these latter effects, which would be incorporated as debits into quality-adjusted life expectancy, were considered small relative to the other factors affecting the quality of life and were therefore ignored.

PROBLEMS IN ASSESSING THE IMPACT OF SIDE EFFECTS

One of the most perplexing problems in assessing the impact of drug side effects is the fact that most existing data are inadequate. Generally, control groups are lacking in studies that have been done. In addition, most attempts to quantify side effects are made during trials before or soon after drugs first appear on the market, involve small groups of patients, and focus on severe or objective rather than mild or subjective reactions. Long-term effects are seldom studied systematically and usually appear in the form of sporadic case reports.

Subjective side effects pose a special problem for the physician and for the policy maker. It is often extremely difficult for the physician to ascertain their presence, or if present, to gauge their intensity. Because human beings are often highly suggestible, the very questioning of a patient about a subjective side effect may increase its likelihood or, if already present, the intensity with which it is experienced. It then becomes difficult to assess whether the expressed morbidity can be entirely attributed to the drug or must be partially attributed to the physician–patient interaction. The physician is confronted with this problem in deciding whether or how to warn a patient about the possibility of subjective side effects. Likewise, the policy maker must decide how to value such effects as a cost of drug therapy. One possible method is demonstrated in chapter 2.

Though most drug side effects occur soon after beginning treatment, some may have long latent periods before manifesting their consequences. The recent description of a possible link between reserpine use and breast cancer exemplifies the problem [Boston Collaborative Drug Surveillance Program, 1974; Armstrong, Stevens, and Doll, 1974; Heinonen et al., 1974]. Other similar relationships, including genetic effects, may yet be discovered. Some drugs have not been in use long enough for the consequences of their long-term use to be fully known.

Physicians, in caring for patients, evaluate their responses to medications and balance these against the severity of side effects for the purpose of optimizing treatment strategies. By sequentially adjusting drugs and dosages, efforts are made to identify regimens that minimize patients' discomfort while achieving the desired decrements in blood pressure. Reversible effects can often be eliminated by changing drug regimens. Irreversible effects, by definition, however, cannot be ameliorated. An analysis cannot fully recreate this flexibility in modeling the impact of drug side effects. The result is an overestimate of the expected costs of drug side effects, the bias being greater for reversible than for irreversible effects.

All of these problems interfere with analytic precision and must be fully recognized, but they do not invalidate the results of analysis. Assumptions are made where data are insufficient or where the natural history of an objective side effect, including its reversibility, is not clear. These allow available information to be used to formulate reasonable approximations of how the drugs in question behave. Where the results of the analysis seem sensitive to particular assumptions, these are examined more closely. Where, on the other hand, the impact of drug side effects is small regardless of the underlying assumptions, results can be accepted with confidence. What follows is simply an effort to push existing knowledge as far as it will take us, an enterprise that every responsible clinician undertakes every time he makes a diagnostic decision and signs his name to a prescription.

ASSUMPTIONS MADE IN EVALUATING THE SIDE EFFECTS OF ANTIHYPERTENSIVE DRUG REGIMENS

The ensuing discussion is limited to three antihypertensive regimens: diuretics (thiazides) alone, diuretics in combination with reserpine, and diuretics in combination with methyldopa. These drugs were chosen because they are in common use and are relatively inexpensive. More complicated regimens are required in only a minority of patients. Furthermore, the analysis is limited by age to a cohort of men and women of 35 through 44 years, and by blood pressure to those with mild (95 through 104 mm Hg) and moderate (105 through 114 mm Hg) hypertension. This age group was selected because it demonstrates a relatively high and rising prevalence of hypertension, and because its members will live long enough to permit side effects to become fully manifest. Mild hypertension was chosen because it includes 70 to 80 percent of all hypertensives and because such patients are at the least risk of cardiovascular disease and, therefore, stand to gain the least from therapy. Prospective studies indicate that the benefits of reduced morbidity and mortality that result from treating severe hypertension are sufficiently large to leave little dispute over the net efficacy of treatment [Veterans Administration Cooperative Study Group, 1967]. A good deal more controversy exists over whether treatment of mild hypertension will produce net benefits, however.

The first assumption underlying the ensuing analysis is that patients adhere to medical regimens and discontinue their medications only when instructed to do so by their physicians. This is not an accurate description of patient behavior, but it simplifies the analysis.[3] Second, it was assumed that, once started, drugs are continued for the lifetime of the patient unless an objective medical indication for discontinuation arises. Though this simplification robs the patient and physician of the therapeutic flexibility discussed previously, it obviates the complex task of simulating the consequences over time of the sequential removal and addition of drugs. Finally, it was assumed that the drugs are used in the dosages described in table 3.1, including chlorothiazide at 1,000 mg per day, reserpine at 0.25 mg per day, and methyldopa at 500 mg per day.

Side effects most commonly associated with these agents are listed in table 3.2. The division of these into "moderate or mild" and "severe" is arbitrary. Many, such as fatigue, depression, headache, and appetite loss, are obviously subjective in nature. In contrast, the presence of fever, anemia, ulcer, or breast cancer can be verified objectively.

DIURETICS

Diuretics, specifically thiazide diuretics, reduce blood pressure by depleting the body of salt and water and, perhaps, by dilating blood vessels as well. They frequently cause side effects, but these are generally mild or even asymptomatic. Serious or life-threatening reactions are rare, and generally these are considered to be relatively safe drugs. Table 3.3 lists major thiazide side effects, their probabilities of occurrence, and increments in expected costs associated with them. Table 3.6 gives estimates of the increase in age-specific mortality for patients commencing therapy at age 40.

HYPOKALEMIA (LOW SERUM POTASSIUM). Diuretic therapy causes the body to excrete excessive amounts of a vital body constituent, potassium ion, which in 25 to 40 percent of patients leads to a reduction in the concentration of serum potassium [Leemhuis and Struyvenberg, 1973; Veterans Administration Cooperative Study Group, 1972; Manner, Brechbill, and Dewitt, 1972]. This can cause subjective symptoms of weakness and muscle fatigue (witness the experience of our British physician whose muscle weakness was relieved by orange juice, a drink containing large amounts of potassium ion) and can lead

---

3. See chapter 4 for discussion and analysis of the problems of adherence and for cost-effectiveness estimates in the presence of incomplete adherence.

Table 3.2: Side effects of antihypertensive drugs.

Drug	Side effects	
	Severe[a]	Moderate or mild[b]
Diuretic	hypokalemia hyperglycemia hyperuricemia dehydration pancreatitis vasculitis blood dyscrasia pulmonary edema	appetite loss nausea constipation diarrhea skin rash photosensitivity fatigue
Reserpine	depression peptic ulcer breast cancer impotence parkinsonism	diarrhea blurring of vision sleepiness dry mouth nasal congestion gynecomastia headache nightmares fatigue edema
Alpha-methyldopa	fever anemia hepatic dysfunction sexual dysfunction parkinsonism blood dyscrasia	sedation depression diarrhea constipation postural hypotension skin rash dry mouth nasal congestion edema weakness non-puerperal lactation

[a] Capable of causing hospitalization or severe emotional anguish, in some cases, death.
[b] Bothersome or uncomfortable; capable of restricting normal activities.

to disturbances in heart rhythms (arrhythmias), especially in persons with underlying heart disease being treated with digitalis [Leemhuis and Struyvenberg, 1973]. Arrhythmias may require hospitalization, and may cause sudden death.

In this analysis it was assumed that serum potassium is normally distributed in the population and that a level less than 3.5 mEq/L is two standard deviations from the mean. This implies that 2.5 percent of the normal population have serum potassium levels below 3.5 mEq/L, as compared with an estimated 33 percent of those receiving diuretics [Leemhuis and Struyvenberg, 1973]. Hence 30 percent of patients develop hypokalemia as a result of diuretic ingestion. Because potassium depletion can

Table 3.3: Estimates of incremental probabilities (P) of experiencing diuretic (D) side effects (SE) and associated morbid events (ME), and their expected annual dollar costs.

Side effect	$P(SE\|D)$	$P(SE\|\overline{D})$	Lifetime increment $\Delta P(SE\|D)$	Morbid event[a]	Annual $P(ME\|SE)$	Annual increment $\Delta P(ME\|D)$[b]	P(Hospitalized|ME)	Cost per hospitalization[c]	Other costs[d]	Annual incremental costs[e]
Hypokalemia	0.33	0.03f	0.15g	arrhythmia	0.001	0.0002	0.25	$2,760l	$175	$0.17
Hyperuricemia				gouty attack						
Males	.41h	.03f	.38		.012	.005k	.001	900m	175p	0.88q
Females	.23h	.03f	.20		.012	.002k	.001	900m	175p	0.35q
Altered glucose tolerance	.21i	.00i	.21	symptomatic hyperglycemia	.01	.002	.20	1,950n	60	0.90
Miscellaneous[j]				miscellaneous						
Upper bound	—	—	—		—	.02	.05	1,550o	100	3.55r
Conservative	—	—	—		—	.005	.05	1,550o	100	0.89r

a Illness to which the patient is predisposed by the side effect.
b Equals $\Delta P(SE\|D) \times P(ME\|SE)$.

c Average disease-specific costs for hospitalized patients in New England [Jones et al., 1975], corrected for inflation from 1970 to 1975 at 15% per year. A single hospitalization was assumed for each illness, recurrences being prevented by adjunctive therapy.

d Approximate incremental costs per morbid event other than those associated with hospitalization (i.e., for physician visits, laboratory tests, medications, etc.). (See note p below for exception.)

e Equals $\Delta P(ME|D) \times [P(\text{Hospitalized}|ME) \times (\text{Cost per hospitalization}) + (\text{Other costs})]$. (For exceptions, see note q below).

f Proportion of normals more than two standard deviations from the mean, rounded to two decimal places.

g Assumes half of hypokalemia is corrected by oral potassium supplements.

h Proportion of patients taking diuretics with uric acid more than two standard deviations above mean for sex.

i Probability that glucose tolerance is altered by diuretic therapy. Assumes that 25% of hypertensives are diabetic or prediabetic, that 86% of these experience altered glucose tolerance, and that no nondiabetics experience this effect.

j Alternative assumptions for the incremental incidences of miscellaneous side effects.

k An upper bound assumption that applies to each year of life.

l Average cost of hospitalization for coronary heart disease [Jones et al., 1975].

m Average cost of hospitalization for "synovitis, bursitis, and tenosynovitis" [Jones et al., 1975].

n Average cost of hospitalization for diabetes mellitus [Jones et al., 1975].

o Average cost of hospitalization for all causes [Jones et al., 1975].

p Applies each year following the first attack of gout. Represents the cost of preventive treatment while the diuretic is continued.

q Expected annual cost due to incident cases. This must be added to $0.87 and $0.35 for men and women, respectively, to account for the on-going annual costs of treatment for cases incident in previous years. (See note p above.)

r Assumed to apply only for the first two years of therapy.

be corrected through the administration of oral potassium supplements, it was further assumed that hypokalemia is corrected
in one-half of depleted patients [Taylor, 1975]. The net incremental probability of hypokalemia is therefore 0.15. In those not
receiving potassium supplements hypokalemia persists as long as
the drug is administered [Leemhuis and Struyvenberg, 1973;
Edmonds and Jasani, 1972].

The probability of nonfatal detected cardiac arrhythmias and
severe muscle weakness was assumed to be increased by 0.001
per year, one-quarter of these requiring hospitalization. Finally,
the rate of sudden death was arbitrarily assumed to be increased
by 10 percent among hypertensives taking diuretics.

HYPERURICEMIA (ELEVATED SERUM URIC ACID). For reasons
that are still controversial, diuretics raise the circulating blood
level of another serum constituent, uric acid. Deposition of uric
acid in body tissues is responsible for a form of arthritis known
as gout. Some physicians consider a gouty attack an indication
for withdrawing diuretics and substituting alternative therapy.
Others treat patients with additional medications that lower serum
uric acid levels. Both methods are effective. Even if untreated,
however, gout only rarely leads to hospitalization and is not
generally believed to cause death.

Increase in serum uric acid to levels greater than two standard
deviations above the mean has been reported to occur in 41 percent of males and 23 percent of females taking thiazides [Bryant
et al., 1962]. Using evidence from the Framingham population
that the prevalence of gout among individuals with elevated uric
acid levels was 19 percent compared with 2.2 percent for those
with normal levels, annual incidence rates of 13.5 and 1.5 per
thousand respectively were calculated by assuming that all
prevalent cases developed during the 14-year period of follow-up
[Hall et al., 1967]. The incremental probability of gout associated
with hyperuricemia would therefore be 12 per thousand, or
0.012. Combining this estimate with the data on diuretic effects
of serum uric acids, an annual incremental probability of developing a first gouty attack would be 0.005 in males and 0.002 in
females. An alternative, more conservative, assumption holds
that this incremental incidence of a first attack is operative only
for the first five years of treatment.

To simplify the analysis it was assumed that the diuretic is
continued and that recurrent attacks of gout are successfully

prevented by adjunctive therapy at a cost of $175 per year. The unusual case of a patient with gout requiring hospitalization was assumed to occur with a probability of one per thousand (0.001) incident cases.

Recent data suggest that hyperuricemia does not contribute to kidney failure [Berger and Yu, 1975]. This potential side effect of diuretic-induced hyperuricemia was not, therefore, considered in the analysis.

HYPERGLYCEMIA (ELEVATED BLOOD SUGAR). Diuretics cause an increase in the circulating concentration of still another blood constituent, blood sugar or glucose, especially in patients with known or incipient diabetes. In one study, the tolerance of diabetics for ingested glucose was diminished in 86 percent of those taking the drug [Shapiro, Benedek, and Small, 1961]. This effect seems to be completely reversible if the offending agent is withdrawn. Some physicians, however, continue the drug so long as the physiological alteration does not produce symptoms. The assumption was made that this practice is observed and that the drug is withdrawn only if a patient develops symptoms of hyperglycemia.

The incremental probability of diuretic-induced symptomatic hyperglycemia was estimated arbitrarily to be 0.01 for patients with abnormal glucose tolerance. Together with the estimates that about 25 percent of hypertensives have diabetes or prediabetes [Kohner et al., 1971] and that 86 percent of these experience altered glucose tolerance [Shapiro, Benedek, and Small, 1961], the incremental annual probability of diuretic-induced symptomatic hyperglycemia is approximately 0.002. Such patients were assumed to have a 20 percent chance of being hospitalized.

As a cause of death, diuretic-induced hyperglycemia is probably negligible and is subsumed under miscellaneous side effects.

MISCELLANEOUS SIDE EFFECTS. Diuretic agents have been associated with the development of a number of rare problems, some clearly linked to the drug, others less so. Among these are various allergic reactions ranging from skin rashes to life-threatening anaphylactic responses. Other rare side effects include various diseases of the blood and inflammatory diseases of blood vessels.

In a fifteen-month prospective study of patients taking chlorothiazide, it was found that roughly 2 percent experienced these reactions [Dinon, Kim, and Vander Veer, 1958]. The upper bound on the incremental annual probability of miscellaneous side effects was therefore taken to be 0.02. This is contrasted with a less pessimistic estimate of 0.005. It was also assumed that these side effects generally abate after withdrawal of the drug, that they occur within the first two years of therapy, and that the probability of hospitalization given one of these untoward responses to a diuretic is 0.05.

Mortality from these effects, which includes that resulting from diuretic-induced hyperglycemia, was arbitrarily assumed to result in an increment of 3 deaths per 100,000 per year at age 50 or, less pessimistically, 1 death per 100,000 per year.

RESERPINE

Reserpine is an antihypertensive agent of about the same potency as diuretics. It lowers blood pressure by inhibiting nerve transmission and thereby reducing constriction of blood vessels. The drug has been in clinical use for many years and has both advocates and opponents among physicians. Its low cost and convenience of administration (once daily) are strong arguments in its favor, while its relatively high incidence of troublesome side effects, especially its tendency to produce depression, detract from its popularity. More recently a pall has been cast over its use by reports of its possible association with breast cancer. Where this debate will end is not yet clear.

Major reserpine side effects and estimates of the incremental probabilities of their occurrence, and increments in expected costs associated with these, are shown in table 3.4. Estimates of the increase in age-specific mortality for patients commencing drug ingestion at age 40 are shown in table 3.6.

DEPRESSION.   Until the recent suggestion that reserpine might be associated with the development of breast cancer, depression was the most widely cited and widely feared consequence of its administration. Nevertheless, there is surprisingly little reliable data available on the frequency with which it occurs or on its consequences for the patients affected.

The conflicting data that do exist are extremely difficult to interpret. Criteria used to define depression are either unstated or widely divergent; drug dosages differ widely; and the characteristics of the populations studied vary.

Some studies show virtually no effect [Veterans Administration Cooperative Study Group, 1972; Bernstein and Kaufman, 1960], while others show a significant effect [Quetsch et al., 1959; Smith, Thurm, and Bromer, 1969; Goodwin, Ebert, and Bunney, 1972]. In Quetsch's retrospective study of 387 hypertensive patients, 26 percent of patients taking reserpine developed depression, compared to 5 percent of matched controls. Of patients with a prior history of depression, 55 percent developed symptoms, compared to 20 percent of those with no such history. In the other positive studies the incidences of reserpine-induced depression were 11.3 and 15 percent. In their review of the literature, Goodwin, Ebert, and Bunney [1972] noted that depression is probably rare among patients using less than 0.5 mg of reserpine daily. Data from the Veterans Administration Study [1972] provide support for this hypothesis.

Goodwin, Ebert, and Bunney [1972] further note that "most" depressive reactions occur within two to eight months of the initiation of therapy, and cite one study in which one-third of depressed patients taking reserpine required hospitalization and one-sixth required electroshock therapy. These figures far exceed the clinical impressions of physicians who frequently dispense antihypertensive medications.

In the analysis, the data of Quetsch et al. [1959] were taken as an upper bound estimate. Assuming that physicians screen out patients with past histories of depression, the probability of becoming depressed on reserpine would be roughly four times that of developing depression off the drug, 0.20 compared to 0.05. This is compared with an alternative, perhaps more realistic, assumption of a two-fold increase in the incidence of depression. It was further assumed that all patients who become depressed do so in the first year of therapy, that all drug-induced depressions severe enough to result in hospitalization occur within the first year of therapy, and that patients experiencing these severe reactions are taken off the drug and recover completely. Thus, while patients may be mildly or moderately depressed for as long as they continue to take the drug, there will be no new occurrences of severe drug-related depression after one year.

The depression associated with reserpine varies in severity. If it does not result in hospitalization, it may require other less expensive therapy delivered on an ambulatory basis. The probability that a reserpine-induced depression would result in hos-

Table 3.4: Estimates of incremental probabilities (P) of experiencing reserpine (R) side effects (SE), and the associated increment in expected annual dollar costs.

Side effect	$P(SE\|R)$	$P(SE\|\bar{R})$	Lifetime increment $\Delta P(SE\|R)$	P(Hospitalized$\|SE$)	Cost per hospitalization[a]	Other costs[b]	Annual incremental costs[c]
Depression							
Upper bound[d]	0.20	0.05	0.15	0.10[k]	$1,140[n]	$200[k]	$47.10[k]
Conservative[e]	.10	.05	.05	0.10[k]	1,140[n]	200[k]	15.70[k]
Peptic ulcer							
Males, upper bound[f]	.07	.05	.02	0.02[l]	2,320[o]	200	4.93
Females, upper bound[f]	.03	.02	.01	0.02[l]	2,230[o]	200	2.46
Conservative	—		.00	0.02[l]	2,320[o]	200	0.00
Breast cancer[g]	.09	.03	.06	1.00[m]	3,180[p]	500	various[q]
Sleepiness[h]	.50	.40	.10	—	—	—	—
Impotence[i]	.33	.31	.02	—	—	—	—
Nasal congestion[j]	.05	—	.05	—	—	—	—

a Average disease-specific costs for hospitalized patients in New England [Jones et al., 1975], corrected for inflation from 1970 to 1975 at 15% per year.
b Approximate annual incremental costs other than those associated with hospitalization (i.e., for physician visits, laboratory tests, medications, etc.).

c Equals $\Delta P(SE|R) \times [P(\text{Hospitalized}|SE) \times (\text{Cost per hospitalization}) + (\text{Other costs})]$.

d Assumes depression occurs four times as often with reserpine as without [Quetsch et al., 1959].

e Assumes depression occurs twice as often with reserpine as without.

f Assumes that the prevalence of ulcer among reserpine users is 1.5 times that of nonusers [Veterans Administration Cooperative Study Group, 1970]. Prevalence for nonusers taken for the 45–64 age group [National Center for Health Statistics, 1973b].

g Lifetime incidences $P(SE|R)$ and $P(SE|\bar{R})$ are multiples ($\times 30$) of annual incidence rates for breast cancer assuming that breast cancer incidence is three times normal in reserpine users, and assuming an average additional life expectancy of 30 years in the absence of breast cancer. For age-specific incidence rates of breast cancer see Haagensen [1971].

h Figures are for groups taking diuretic plus reserpine and diuretic only. The controls are therefore not strictly comparable to the general population, though sleepiness is not a commonly reported side effect of diuretic usage [Bulpitt and Dollery, 1973].

i These data do not support reports of impotence as a side effect of reserpine use [Bulpitt and Dollery, 1973]. It is virtually impossible to find reports of the prevalence of impotence in the normal population, but it is almost certainly substantial.

j From McKenney [1974].

k Assumed to apply only in first year after initiation of reserpine therapy.

l Assumed to apply in each year of remaining life.

m Assumes one hospitalization in the first year, and one hospitalization each year from year 5 until death for those not cured in the first year. Assumes that 50% are permanently cured in year 1, 36% die in year 5, and 14% die in year 10, consistent with a 64% five-year survival [Silverberg and Holleb, 1975].

n Average cost of hospitalization for "mental, psychoneurotic, and personality disorders" [Jones et al., 1975].

o Average cost of hospitalization for peptic ulcer disease [Jones et al., 1975].

p Average cost of hospitalization for "malignant and unspecified neoplasms" [Jones et al., 1975].

q The disease is assumed to occur in the tenth year after initiation of therapy. Expected annual incremental costs are $220 in the year the diagnosis is made, $15 in years 2 through 4, $110 in year 5, $30 in years 6 through 10, and zero thereafter. See note m above.

pitalization was arbitrarily set at 10 percent in the first year of therapy, and the ambulatory costs of drugs and psychiatric care for depressed patients were assumed to average $200.

Though there is no direct evidence, it seems likely that reserpine-induced depression may also cause some patients to commit suicide. To relate reserpine use to suicide rates, it was assumed that all patients who commit suicide are depressed, and that depression induced by reserpine is identical to depression induced by other exogenous and endogenous factors. As an upper bound, it was therefore assumed that a population ingesting reserpine can be expected to have a suicide rate four times that of a population of comparable age and sex [Kramer et al., 1972]. The added risk of suicide was assumed to persist for five years. This is contrasted with a more conservative assumption of a doubling of suicide rates among reserpine users.

PEPTIC ULCER DISEASE. Reserpine has been reported to exacerbate preexisting ulcer disease and to precipitate gastrointestinal symptoms in some patients. In large doses, it increases peptic acid secretion [Bachrach, 1959], a phenomenon that could explain those effects. Careful review of the literature, however, reveals an almost total absence of convincing evidence to support ulcerogenic effects in doses used for the treatment of mild essential hypertension [Sleisenger and Fordtran, 1973].

Because of the notoriety that this alleged effect of reserpine has received, however, peptic ulcer is included in the analysis as a potential consequence of the drug's use. Upper bound estimates of the incremental incidence of ulcer were based on fragmentary data from the Veterans Administration Cooperative Study [1970] indicating that ulcer disease and its symptoms occurred roughly 1.5 times as frequently in treated male patients as in the control group. In males aged 45–64, this would mean an increase in the probability of developing an ulcer from 0.05 to 0.07 over the rest of the patient's lifetime. In females the comparable increment would be from 0.02 to 0.03. It was further assumed that patients who develop ulcers do so during the first year of therapy and that ulcers persist after the discontinuation of the drug. Thus, those patients who have developed ulcers because of reserpine use would have the same rates of hospitalization and mortality as those who develop ulcers for other reasons. It was assumed that the annual probability of hospitalization for such patients is 0.02 and that age-specific death rates are 1.5 times higher in patients with ulcer disease than in the general population.

BREAST CANCER. Recent retrospective studies have indicated that breast cancer is 2.0 to 3.9 times as common in women taking reserpine as in matched controls not taking the drug [Boston Collaborative Drug Surveillance Program, 1974; Armstrong, Stevens, and Doll, 1974; Heinonen et al., 1974]. These findings have been challenged by other investigators [Mack et al., 1975; O'Fallon, Labarthe, and Kurland, 1975; Laska et al., 1975]. Nevertheless, they must be taken into account in projecting the potential costs of treating patients with reserpine. The analysis is performed both under the assumption that a tripling of the life-time risk of breast cancer does occur, as suggested by the initial reports, and alternatively, that reserpine use and breast cancer are not associated.

Several other assumptions were made, based on the best available data regarding the natural history of reserpine-induced breast cancer. These are:

• that all reserpine-induced breast cancer occurs exactly ten years after the drug is begun. This assumption, though arbitrary, reflects findings that the incremental probability of developing breast cancer as a result of reserpine use increases with duration of therapy [Boston Collaborative Drug Study, 1974];
• that once the disease has appeared, it follows the same natural history as in patients not taking reserpine;
• that the five-year and ten-year survival rates are 64 percent and 50 percent respectively [Silverberg and Holleb, 1975]. The 50 percent who survive ten years were assumed to be cured in the first year of treatment and to require no subsequent medical services directly attributable to breast cancer;
• that patients with reserpine-induced breast cancer are hospitalized once in the first year and, for those not cured, once in each year from the fifth year following diagnosis until death; and
• that death rates from breast cancer, as well as incidence rates, triple among the cohort taking reserpine, relative to those in the general population [Robbins, 1967], after the initial ten-year latent period.

This treatment of the natural history of breast cancer will probably bias projections of the dollar costs associated with its treatment upward. This is true because many cases would probably occur several years after the ten-year latent period. Moving these expenditures earlier in time increases their contribution to the total, discounted outlays for breast cancer, since the process of discounting lessens the magnitude of expenditures occurring later in time.

METHYLDOPA

Methyldopa, introduced into clinical use in 1960, is a moderately potent antihypertensive agent useful in the treatment of moderate or severe hypertension, usually in conjunction with thiazide diuretics or other drugs. Like reserpine, methyldopa causes a reduction in vascular resistance that results in lowered arterial blood pressure. Relative freedom from serious side effects has contributed to its popularity. Milder untoward effects, especially drowsiness, lethargy, or decrease in mental acuity, are frequent, however, though often transitory. In several studies, these side effects have led to discontinuation of therapy in from 7 to 21 percent of patients [Dollery, 1965; Johnson et al., 1966; Colwill et al., 1964].

Table 3.5 summarizes data on the most frequent and most serious side effects of methyldopa, indicating the incremental probabilities of their occurrence and the medical care costs associated with them. Mortality from any of these side effects is extremely rare and is ignored in the analysis.

HEPATIC DYSFUNCTION. Methyldopa has been demonstrated to cause asymptomatic derangements of liver function in approximately 6 percent of patients and, more rarely, to result in clinical syndromes indistinguishable from viral hepatitis [Elkington, Schreiber, and Conn, 1969]. Usually this disease remits when the drug is withdrawn, but occasional well-documented examples of chronic hepatitis and even fatalities have been reported [Toghill et al., 1974; Rehman, Keith, and Gall, 1973]. In addition, occasional patients have undergone exploratory abdominal surgery because of suspected obstruction of the biliary tract.

In the analysis it was assumed that of the 6 percent of patients who develop abnormalities in liver function tests, 10 percent experience symptomatic episodes of hepatitis. Using the data of Toghill et al. [1974], it was further estimated that 10 percent of patients with acute hepatitis progress to a chronic phase even after drug withdrawal, with an annual treatment cost of $200. These figures are almost certainly upper bound estimates. It was

Table 3.5: Estimates of incremental probabilities (P) of experiencing methyldopa (M) side effects (SE), and the associated increment in expected annual dollar costs.

Side effect	$P(SE\|M)$	$P(SE\|\overline{M})$	Annual increment $\Delta P(SE\|M)$	$P(\text{Hospitalized}\|SE)$	Cost per hospitalization[a]	Other costs	Annual incremental costs[b]
Hepatic dysfunction, symptomatic	0.006[c]	0.001[d]	0.005	.5[j]	$2,420[k]	$200	$6.15[j]
Hemolytic anemia	.0005[e]	—	.0005	.5[j]	1,870[l]	—	0.47[j]
Fever	.015[f]	—	.015	.5[j]	1,550[m]	—	11.60[j]
Drowsiness							
initial	.70[g]	.39[h]	.31	—	—	—	—
persistent	.57[h]	.39[h]	.18	—	—	—	—
Sexual dysfunction	.13[i]	.00	.13	—	—	—	—

[a] Average disease-specific costs for hospitalized patients in New England [Jones et al., 1975], corrected for inflation from 1970 to 1975 at 15% per year.

[b] Equals $\Delta P(SE\|M) \times [P(\text{Hospitalized}\|SE) \times (\text{Cost per hospitalization}) + (\text{Other costs})]$.

[c] Assumes an estimated 6% total incidence of hepatic dysfunction, of which 1 in 10 are symptomatic [Elkington, Schreiber, and Conn, 1969]—almost certainly an upper bound as determined by the relative rarity of verified case reports in the literature.

[d] The annual incidence of hepatitis for 1973, corrected for estimated under-reporting of the disease [Center for Disease Control, 1975a and b].

[e] From Carstairs et al. [1966], and Böttiger and Westerholm [1973].

[f] From Colwill et al. [1964].

[g] From Horwitz et al. [1967].

[h] From Bulpitt and Dollery [1973]. Symptoms were reported on a questionnaire during therapy. Figures are for groups taking thiazides plus methyldopa and thiazides alone. The controls, therefore, are not strictly comparable to the general population, though drowsiness is not a commonly reported side effect of thiazides.

[i] From Newman and Salerno [1974]. Data were obtained from male patients by "close questioning." Controls were on thiazides. The figures used represent adjustment of these data to a 50:50 male:female population and represent an upper bound on the incidence of methyldopa-associated impotence when compared to other reports [Bulpitt and Dollery, 1973].

[j] Assumed to apply only in first year after initiation of methyldopa therapy. The estimated 10% of patients who develop chronic hepatitis contribute insignificantly to expected annual costs and are therefore ignored.

[k] Average cost of hospitalization for "all other digestive diseases" [Jones et al., 1975].

[l] Average cost of hospitalization for "diseases of the blood" [Jones et al., 1975].

[m] Average cost of hospitalization for all causes [Jones et al., 1975].

also assumed that hepatitis, when it occurs, results in a single hospitalization in one-half of patients.

HEMOLYTIC ANEMIA. Methyldopa has been shown to be associated, in 20 percent of treated patients, with the development of a positive direct Coombs test, a hallmark of an autoimmune process affecting red blood cells [Carstairs et al., 1966]. Hemolytic anemia develops in a small proportion of such patients, estimated from adverse drug report data to be about 1 in 6,000 [Worlledge, Carstairs, and Dacie, 1966; Bötliger and Westerholm, 1973]. If only one-third of adverse drug reactions are actually reported, this incidence becomes 1 in 2,000 (0.0005). Both in England and Sweden methyldopa is the most common cause of reported drug-induced hemolytic anemia [Worlledge, Carstairs, and Dacie, 1966; Bötliger and Westerholm, 1973]. Usually this anemia responds promptly to drug withdrawal. Occasional serious episodes of hemolysis have been reported, however, which in rare instances have contributed to the patient's death [Bötliger and Westerholm, 1973]. It was assumed for the analysis that one-half of patients who develop anemia are hospitalized on a single occasion for evaluation and treatment, and that after the diagnosis methyldopa is permanently discontinued.

FEVER. Febrile, flu-like illnesses, frequently associated with liver function abnormalities, have been reported to occur in 1 to 3 percent of patients [Parker, 1974; Glontz and Saslaw, 1968; Klein and Kaminsky, 1973]. These occur within a few days of starting treatment and respond promptly to discontinuation of the drug if the cause is recognized. If not, they may lead to hospitalization and extensive investigations to discover the cause of the fever. It was assumed that one-half of patients who develop fever while receiving methyldopa are hospitalized for evaluation and that thereafter the drug is discontinued.

DROWSINESS. Up to 70 percent of patients complain of drowsiness when they are first started on treatment with methyldopa. In patients who depend upon mental acuity in their work, this may prove especially troublesome. Occasional instances of severe depression have been reported, uniformly in patients with depressive symptoms before taking the drug. Frequently, mild symptoms subside even though treatment with the drug is continued. Because drowsiness is such a subjective symptom, however, it is not known whether the sedative effect of methyldopa really dissipates or whether the patient merely learns to live with his lethargy without complaining.

SEXUAL DYSFUNCTION. Sexual dysfunction is manifest by a diminished interest in sex or, in male patients, in a diminished ability to sustain an erection or ejaculate. Because of the reluctance of patients to reveal such information, evaluation of these effects of drugs depends heavily on the methods employed to obtain data. Results for methyldopa are conflicting. Some studies show a slight or no increase in impotence [Bulpitt and Dollery, 1973] and others a substantial one [Newman and Salerno, 1974].

Impact of Side Effects on Dollar Costs and Mortality

To determine how drug side effects influence the dollar costs and mortality benefits of treating hypertension, it was assumed, for simplicity, that the probabilities of occurrence of side effects are independent of one another. Hence, incremental impacts on costs of treatment and mortality rates can be added together. The magnitudes of these impacts were then assessed relative to the outcomes of treatment itself as derived in chapter 2 for specific age, sex, and blood pressure cohorts. Estimated annual costs of treating essential hypertension in the absence of side effects (table 3.1) serve as reference points in estimating the dollar costs of side effects.

Calculations were performed under alternative assumptions about the level of blood pressure before and after treatment:

Pretreatment	*Posttreatment*
110 mm Hg	90 mm Hg
100 mm Hg	85 mm Hg

To determine the fraction of benefit realized from lowering blood pressure, the age-varying partial benefit assumption was employed. Thus, a treated patient experiences death rates based on a reduction by a fraction of the difference between those associated with pretreatment and posttreatment blood pressures, that fraction varying with the age at initiation of therapy and the duration of treatment (see chapter 2).

IMPACTS ON THE COSTS OF TREATMENT

Tables 3.3, 3.4, and 3.5 show the expected annual increments in per capita costs associated with side effects of diuretics,

Table 3.6: Annual increments to age-specific mortality rates (per 100,000) due to side effects for males and females, 40–74 years old.

Drug	Males				Females			
	40–44	45–54	55–64	65–74	40–44	45–54	55–64	65–74
Diuretic								
Totals								
Upper bound[a]	3.0	4.5	12.0	21.5	1.5	3.0	9.5	19.7
Conservative[b]	1.9	2.2	5.2	8.0	0.4	0.7	2.7	6.2
Reserpine								
Totals								
Upper bound	67.6	4.9	4.9	4.9	24.5	104.7	188.3	303.9
Conservative	31.3	0.0	0.0	0.0	11.2	0.0	0.0	0.0
Depression								
Upper bound[c]	62.7	—	—	—	22.4	—	—	—
Conservative[d]	31.3	—	—	—	11.2	—	—	—
Breast cancer								
Upper bound[e]	—	—	—	—	—	102.6	186.2	301.8
Conservative[e]	—	—	—	—	—	0.0	0.0	0.0
Ulcer								
Upper bound[f]	4.9	4.9	4.9	4.9	2.1	2.1	2.1	2.1
Conservative	0.0	0.0	0.0	0.0	0.0	0.0	0.0	0.0
Reserpine and Diuretic								
Totals								
Upper bound	70.6	9.4	16.9	26.4	26.0	107.7	197.8	323.6
Conservative	33.2	2.2	5.2	8.0	11.6	0.7	2.7	6.2

[a] Includes hypokalemia and miscellaneous side effects including hyperglycemia. Sex- and age-specific rates of sudden death from cardiovascular disease are assumed to be increased by 10% in patients with hypokalemia. Assumes an incremental death rate of 3 per 100,000 at age 50 due to miscellaneous effects.

[b] Assumes incremental death rate of only 1 per 100,000 at age 50 due to miscellaneous effects.

[c] Four times suicide rate for normals for first five years, then no subsequent suicides. Suicide rates are from Kramer et al. [1972].

[d] Two times suicide rate for normals for first five years, then no subsequent suicides.

[e] Assumes a tripling of age-specific death rates from breast cancer, all cases occurring 10 years following initiation of reserpine therapy. See Robbins [1967] for base rates.

[f] Crude death rate for ulcers divided by the prevalence of the disease. Age-specific rates not available.

reserpine, and methyldopa respectively. Both "upper bound" and "conservative" assumptions are given for several side effects. The conservative assumption set, which is probably a more realistic interpretation of the evidence, differs from the upper bound assumptions in that: (1) all attacks of gout occur within the first five years of therapy, (2) the annual incidence of miscellaneous side effects requiring hospitalization is only 1 in 200, rather than 1 in 50, (3) depression has only twice, rather than four times, the incidence with reserpine as without, (4) ulcer is not a side effect of reserpine, and (5) breast cancer is not caused by reserpine use.

Expected lifetime costs (discounted at 5 percent per annum) associated with the treatment of side effects for 40-year-old patients with mild hypertension are shown in table 3.7. These are combined with lifetime costs of antihypertensive treatment (table 3.1), to arrive at the total present-value lifetime costs with and without side effects (table 3.8).

If the conservative assumption set were considered to be three times as likely as the upper bound assumption set, and the

Table 3.7: Expected increments to discounted (at 5 percent per year) lifetime dollar costs associated with drug-related morbid events for 40-year-old patients with mild hypertension (95–104 mm Hg).

	Upper bound assumptions		Conservative assumptions	
Side effect	Males	Females	Males	Females
Thiazide diuretic				
Hypokalemia	$ 3	$ 3	$ 3	$ 3
Hyperuricemia	163	65	60	24
Hyperglycemia	14	14	14	14
Miscellaneous	7	7	2	2
Total	187	89	79	43
Reserpine				
Depression	47	47	16	16
Ulcer	77	39	0	0
Breast cancer	0	264	0	0
Total	124	350	16	16
Methyldopa				
Hepatitis	8	8	8	8
Anemia	1	1	1	1
Fever	12	12	12	12
Total	21	21	21	21
Diuretic + reserpine				
Total	311	439	95	59
Diuretic + methyldopa				
Total	208	110	100	64

Table 3.8: Expected discounted (at 5 percent per year) lifetime treatment costs with and without drug side effects.

Drug	With side effects		Without side effects
	Upper bound	Conservative	
Diuretic + reserpine			
Males	$3,190	$2,970	$2,880
Females	3,580	3,200	3,140
Diuretic + methyldopa			
Males	4,210	4,100	4,000
Females	4,490	4,440	4,380

diuretic-plus-reserpine regimen and the diuretic-plus-methyldopa regimen were equally prevalent, then the expected incremental lifetime cost due to drug side effects would be $138 for men and $115 for women. This is the basis for the $125 figure used in chapter 2.

The following points emerge from tables 3.7 and 3.8:

• Even under the upper bound assumptions, the expected costs associated with diuretic side effects add only about 2 to 6 percent to the total lifetime costs of treatment.

• Under upper bound assumptions for the combined regimen of a diuretic and reserpine, side effects increase the incremental lifetime costs of treatment by 11 to 14 percent. Under the conservative assumptions, which reduce the incidence of depression, exclude breast cancer and ulcer, and limit the incidence of gout to five years, this figure falls to 2 to 3 percent. For women, 70 percent of this difference is due to the exclusion of breast cancer.

• Methyldopa side effects add less than 1 percent to treatment costs.

It should be noted that all of these figures are expected costs, in that the dollar costs of each side effect are weighted by their respective probabilities of occurrence. If individuals had to pay these costs, this would be an underestimate of true cost, because risk-averse individuals would be willing to pay more than the expected cost to avoid low-probability risks of catastrophically high costs such as those of treating breast cancer. Since treatments for most of the drug side effects considered here are usually covered by health insurance, however, the individual need not pay this additional risk premium. From the viewpoint of society (and fiscal intermediaries), expected cost is the appropriate measure.

IMPACT OF DRUG SIDE EFFECTS ON LIFE EXPECTANCY

Table 3.6 shows the increments to age-specific mortality rates associated with the major side effects. Using the model described in chapter 2, net changes in life expectancy and quality-adjusted life expectancy (that is, life expectancy augmented by improvements in quality of life due to prevention of stroke and myocardial infarction and diminished by adverse subjective side effects) associated with blood pressure control were calculated for 40-year-olds (35–44) with pretreatment diastolic blood pressures of 100 mm Hg and 110 mm Hg. The calculations were made under the age-varying partial benefit assumption, with discounting at 5 percent per year, and under both the upper bound and conservative assumptions about drug side effects. The results are given in table 3.9 for the regimen of diuretic plus reserpine. Mortality from methyldopa was assumed to be zero. Observations from these results are as follows:

• For reserpine, breast cancer is by far the most important potential cause of reduced life expectancy. If estimates of the

Table 3.9: Net increase in life expectancy and quality-adjusted life expectancy from blood pressure control for 40-year-olds, under various assumptions regarding drug side effects for a regimen of diuretic plus reserpine.

Sex	Pre-treatment diastolic blood pressure (mm Hg)	No mortal side effects	Upper bound including breast cancer	Upper bound excluding breast cancer	Con-servative
		Change in life expectancy			
M	100	0.46	0.40	0.40	0.44
M	110	.66	.61	.61	.65
F	100	.44	.20	.41	.43
F	110	.59	.35	.56	.58
		Change in quality-adjusted life expectancy			
M	100	0.34	0.28	0.28	0.32
M	110	.57	.52	.52	.56
F	100	.33	.09	.30	.32
F	110	.51	.27	.48	.50

Assumes: age-varying partial benefit; discounting at 5% per annum; stepped blood pressure control.

association between reserpine and breast cancer are true, the life-prolonging benefits of therapy would be significantly reduced for women, by 70 percent and 50 percent respectively, for diastolic blood pressures of 100 mm Hg (95–104 mm Hg) and 110 mm Hg (105–114 mm Hg). These trends would be even stronger if the effects of breast cancer on the quality of life were taken into account. Compared to breast cancer, the expected impacts of other side effects of reserpine on the life expectancy benefits of antihypertensive treatment in women are very small.

• For males, depression is the largest single contributor to reduced life expectancy benefit for reserpine, accounting for about half of the difference between the expected benefit with side effects and the expected benefit without. The importance of this effect derives from the higher suicide rate in males. All side effects together, however, reduce life expectancy by at most 15 or 20 percent.

• The expected impacts of diuretic- and methyldopa-related side effects on mortality are very small in both men and women.

IMPACT OF DRUG SIDE EFFECTS ON THE COST-EFFECTIVENESS OF ANTIHYPERTENSIVE THERAPY

The overall impact of objective drug side effects on cost-effectiveness of therapy is found by incorporating their mortality and costs into the cost-effectiveness calculations described in chapter 2. The resulting measures of net dollar cost per year of increased quality-adjusted life expectancy reflect the relative efficiency of antihypertensive treatment under various assumptions about side effects. As in chapter 2, subjective side effects were taken into account by assuming a loss in quality of life equivalent to some fraction of years lived. For diuretic plus reserpine, this fraction was taken to be 1 percent; for diuretic plus methyldopa, this fraction was taken to be 1.25 percent, reflecting a slightly higher incidence of subjective side effects with methyldopa. The results are given in table 3.10.

The following conclusions may be drawn:

• The potential impact of reserpine-induced breast cancer on the cost-effectiveness of treating mild and moderate hypertension is substantial and deserves close attention in future research.

• In males, the cost-effectiveness of reserpine use is moderately

Table 3.10: The impact of objective and subjective drug side effects on the cost-effectiveness of treatment for 40-year-olds with mild and moderate hypertension.

Sex	Pretreatment diastolic blood pressure (mm Hg)	No side effects	Subjective side effects only[a]	Upper bound objective side effects[b]		Conservative objective side effects[b]
				Including breast cancer	Excluding breast cancer	
			Diuretic plus reserpine			
M	100	$5,750	$8,280	$11,100	$11,100	$9,070
M	110	3,720	4,630	5,650	5,650	4,880
F	100	5,950	8,840	36,480	10,270	9,290
F	110	4,050	5,320	11,410	6,000	5,540
			Diuretic plus methyldopa			
M	100	$8,040	$13,130	$13,830		$13,470
M	110	5,250	7,040	7,430		7,230
F	100	8,470	14,310	14,690		14,530
F	110	5,870	8,360	8,600		8,500

Assumes: age-varying partial benefit; discounting at 5% per annum; stepped blood pressure control.

[a] For the reserpine regimen, subjective side effects are assumed to diminish the quality of life by an amount equivalent to 1 percent of remaining present-value life years (as in chapter 2). For the methyldopa regimen, subjective side effects are assumed to diminish the quality of life by an amount equivalent to 1.25 percent of remaining present-value life years.

[b] Cost-effectiveness is defined as: (Cost of treatment − Savings from cardiovascular morbidity + Cost of medical care in added years of life + Cost of treating objective drug side effects) / (Increase in life expectancy adjusted for mortal side effects + Adjustment for reduction in cardiovascular morbidity − Adjustment for subjective side effects).

sensitive to assumptions concerning the incidence, severity, and consequences of depression.

• Differences in cost and subjective side effects between drug regimens have a substantial impact on cost-effectiveness, outweighing differences in objective side effects.

Close attention to the impact of side effects, subjective and objective, is indicated in prospective studies of blood pressure treatment, with particular emphasis on those identified by this analysis to be significant.

Antihypertensive Medications in Perspective

This review of the impact of untoward responses to antihypertensive medications on the costs and benefits of treatment has emphasized the ways in which those drugs detract from net benefits. Though it is always important for physicians and policy makers to keep in mind the risks incurred in any pharmacological intervention, a few comments are necessary to balance the perspective of this chapter.

First, this discussion has been limited to patients with mild and moderate diastolic hypertension. The assessment of the net benefits of drug therapy set forth above cannot, therefore, be taken to apply to more severe forms of hypertension, which may require higher doses or more potent medication to achieve blood pressure control with attendant higher risks of untoward responses. On the other hand, control can be expected to confer greater benefits in such patients.

Second, only three basic blood pressure regimens have been dealt with. The diuretic-plus-reserpine combination may well present antihypertensive therapy in its worst light with regard to the impact of treatment side effects on death rates. Other antihypertensive agents including alpha-methyldopa, which is at least as popular as reserpine, seem to have significantly fewer potentially fatal side effects. Certainly, no other drug has known effects comparable to the possible association of reserpine with breast cancer in women.

Third, reserpine has virtues that have not been sufficiently emphasized: (a) It is, as table 3.1 indicates, the least expensive of the antihypertensive medications by a substantial margin. Alpha-methyldopa therapy is at least 3.4 times as costly, which means an incremental, discounted lifetime expenditure of approximately $800 per person. The combination of hydralazine and propranolol is 8.4 times as expensive, for an incremental expenditure of at least $2,000 per patient. (b) Reserpine's pharmacological characteristics permit the drug to be taken once daily, rather than several times daily as in the case of most other medications. Adherence to therapy and hence expected benefits are thereby likely to be increased. (c) There is less uncertainty about the long-term consequences of reserpine use than of other medications. One reason is that reserpine has been in use longer than most other antihypertensive drugs. Knowledge that reserpine may increase the incidence of breast cancer prejudices us against its use in women. Other medications may have equally disastrous consequences that have simply not yet come to light. (d) There is some evidence that reserpine may have fewer subjective side effects among chronic users than other drugs. Bulpitt and Dollery concluded that "the widespread practice of treating mild hypertension with a diuretic ± reserpine would appear to be justified by the paucity of side effects" [Bulpitt and Dollery, 1973]. These authors found that the average total complaint rate (total number of complaints divided by number of patients) was the same for a diuretic alone and for a diuretic with reserpine, and was lower in males for this drug regimen than for alpha-methyldopa with a diuretic. In females there was little difference. Given the sensitivity of cost-effectiveness to the importance of subjective side effects (figure 2.18), these effects, and costs, may well make reserpine plus a diuretic a more cost-effective regimen than methyldopa plus a diuretic, despite the risks of the former. The estimates in table 3.10, in which the subjective side effects of methyldopa were assumed to be 25 percent greater than those of reserpine, support this hypothesis. This conclusion cannot be made more definitive until comparative data on subjective side effects of these drugs are available.

Finally, the impact of side effects on adherence to therapy has not been discussed. Both simplicity of the regimen and freedom from side effects would be expected to improve the rate of adherence. Hence, an indirect cost of side effects is the extent to which they discourage the use of medications. An alternative viewpoint is that nonadherence reflects the patient's judgment that the costs of therapy outweigh the benefits, but it is questionable whether the patient is fully enough informed to make such decisions rationally.

There is little doubt that people are better off without high blood pressure than with it. On the other hand, treatment of hypertension, as the British physician quoted at the outset of this chapter would testify, can make a patient who initially felt well feel awful. It is not clear a priori that an iatrogenic disease is better than a natural one.

4. Obstacles to Controlling Hypertension

The cost-effectiveness of antihypertensive treatment depends not only on its inherent efficacy but also on the degree to which it can be successfully applied in practice. Unfortunately, serious obstacles to initiating and maintaining effective treatment once the patient is aware of the condition exist; these have a substantial impact on the cost-effectiveness of that treatment. The ability to achieve blood pressure control in patients with established hypertension depends on whether or not treatment is prescribed and, if prescribed, on whether it is successful in controlling blood pressure to the degree desired. Further, it depends importantly on whether patients remain under continuous medical care and, if they do, on the degree to which they adhere to prescribed regimens.

Failure to Initiate Treatment

The failure of patients to obtain treatment for hypertension despite awareness of its existence may result either from their failure to seek care or from the reluctance of physicians to initiate therapy. Regardless of cause, a recent national survey indicated that fully 25 percent of patients who were aware of their hypertension never received treatment for it [Harris, 1973]. Because hypertension is frequently asymptomatic, and because the risk of increased morbidity and mortality conferred by it are in the future, it is often not perceived to be a problem requiring urgent attention. Barriers to receiving care and the inconvenience and cost of treatment become especially critical under these circumstances.

To heighten public awareness of the seriousness of hyperten-

Note: The authors of this chapter are William B. Stason, Milton C. Weinstein, and Donald S. Shepard.

111

sion and to stress the importance of having one's blood pressure monitored and, if necessary, treated, extensive multimedia campaigns have been sponsored by the National High Blood Pressure Education Program and by the American Heart Association. It is too early to know what impact these have had. Other approaches have focused on facilitating access to health care, either by improving referral from screening sites [Finnerty, Shaw, and Himmelsbach, 1973; Charman, 1974] or by providing care close to the screening site [Alderman and Schoenbaum, 1975; Sackett et al., 1975]. These efforts appear to have been remarkably successful, at least in achieving initiation of treatment.

Providers, too, must share responsibility for the failure of many hypertensives to receive treatment. Uncertainty about the efficacy of treatment and lack of enthusiasm for managing hypertension are both involved. In one study, for example, only one-half of hypertensive patients admitted to the hospital for unrelated surgical procedures were receiving treatment at the time of admission despite the fact that nearly all had been seen by their private physicians within the preceding three months [Langfeld, 1973]. Other studies confirm problems with provider behavior [Frohlich et al., 1971; Aronow, Allen, and De Cristofaro, 1975].

Undoubtedly, the lack of definitive evidence for the efficacy of treating mild hypertensives underlies much of the reluctance of physicians to treat these patients. The National High Blood Pressure Education Program recognizes this situation by recommending that treatment with antihypertensive medications be optional for diastolic pressures less than 105 mm Hg [National High Blood Pressure Education Program, 1973b]. Until uncertainties about the benefits of treatment relative to its side effects and costs are resolved, physicians will, justifiably, remain ambivalent about whether to treat mild hypertensives. It is hoped that clinical trials such as the federally funded Hypertension Detection and Follow-up Program will help to resolve this problem.

Doubts regarding the efficacy of treatment cannot, however, account for the observed failure to initiate treatment in patients with moderate and severe hypertension, nor can it account for the reluctance to prescribe medications in doses adequate to achieve the desired degree of blood pressure control or for the failure to monitor on a regular basis patients with borderline or mild hypertension who are not under treatment. Because such minor elevations in blood pressure increase the risk of cardiovascular complications and predispose to further elevations in blood pressure to levels for which treatment is unquestionably valuable [Miall and Chinn, 1974], continued follow-up of these patients has been unequivocally recommended even if therapy is not prescribed [National High Blood Pressure Education Program, 1973b]. Educational programs to disseminate current information and to encourage interest in the management of hypertension is critical to any strategy aimed at achieving improved effectiveness of blood pressure control.

Failure of Prescribed Treatment to Achieve Blood Pressure Control

The failure of prescribed antihypertensive treatment to achieve blood pressure control may result from pharmacological resistance, from inadequate prescription practices by physicians, or, most importantly, from incomplete adherence by patients to prescribed regimens. Each or all may be involved in any individual case, and it is frequently difficult to ascertain the primary culprit. That treatment failure is a major problem, however, is clearly indicated by the fact that only half of hypertensives on medications have their blood pressures "in control" [Wilber and Barrow, 1972; Schoenberger et al., 1972; Borhani and Borkman, 1968; National High Blood Pressure Education Program, 1973e].

PHARMACOLOGICAL RESISTANCE

Pharmacological resistance refers to the inability of medications to achieve blood pressure control even when taken regularly. Resistance is usually a relative rather than absolute phenomenon. With medications currently available a patient's blood pressure can almost always be lowered to some degree but frequently not to normal levels. Because the incidence and severity of medication side effects are often related to dosage and drug type, from a practical point of view the optimal regimen may reflect a tradeoff between achieving the desired lowering of blood pressure and a tolerable level of side effects.

The extent to which pharmacological resistance impedes the effective control of blood pressure is difficult to estimate because distinguishing it from inadequate prescription practices or incomplete adherence is a problem. But when maximal efforts to achieve blood pressure control have been attempted in clinical trials, normalization of blood pressure has resulted in the large majority of patients [Veterans Administration Cooperative Study Group, 1967, 1970; Taylor, 1975; Stamler et al., 1975]. Hence pharmacological resistance seems to account for only a small proportion of treatment failures, and, even in these, careful adjustment of drug type and dosage can frequently achieve desired blood pressure control. When unusual resistance is encountered, the possibility of a secondary form of hypertension, possibly amenable to specific surgical interventions, must be considered. Future research to develop medications that are both more effective and less likely to produce undesirable side effects will undoubtedly further mitigate the problem of pharmacological resistance.

INADEQUATE PRESCRIPTION PRACTICES

Inadequate prescription practices must be recognized as a contributing cause of failures to achieve blood pressure control. The physician's attitudes toward the treatment of hypertension, his knowledge of alternative drug regimens, and his ability to encourage adherence to adjunctive therapies such as weight loss or salt restriction are all involved. It is evident from the expressed lack of enthusiasm of many physicians for managing and treating chronic and asymptomatic problems such as hypertension that changes in physician behavior are vital in any efforts to improve the effectiveness of blood pressure control.

PROBLEMS WITH ADHERENCE

Problems with adherence to medical regimens are both widespread and complex. Two separate but related dimensions exist. The first is the failure of the patient to remain under continuous medical care, the so-called dropout problem. The second is the inability or unwillingness of the patient to adhere to a prescribed treatment that, in addition to medications, may include changes in diet, physical activity, and lifestyle. Both underconsumption and overconsumption of medications may be involved. The root cause may derive either from a lack of understanding of the regimen or from a lack of motivation to adhere to it.

The cost-effectiveness and, ultimately, policy implications of these two problems are very different. A dropout from medical care fails to receive the benefits of treatment but, at the same time, does not incur costs or utilize health care resources. On the other hand, a patient who remains in care but fails to adhere faithfully to a medical regimen usually consumes a disproportionate share of resources relative to the health benefits received. The cost-effectiveness of treatment is commensurately reduced.

Though conceptual distinctions should be clearly drawn between the dropout problem and that of poor adherence to medical regimens, they will be considered together here under the rubric "adherence." The reason for this is the overlap that exists with regard both to causal or predisposing factors and to approaches taken to their solutions. (See chapter 6 for analysis and policy implications in which they are considered separately.)

Without doubt, failure to adhere seriously compromises the effectiveness of antihypertensive treatment. Population surveys have indicated that 29 to 50 percent of known hypertensives were not taking medications at all [Wilber and Barrow, 1972; Schoenberger et al., 1972; Harris, 1973; Borhani and Borkman, 1968]. These percentages include both patients who were never treated and those in whom treatment had been discontinued. In the Harris survey [1973], major reasons given for discontinuing treatment once begun were "advice of the physician" (54 percent) and the patient's belief that he or she "didn't need it any more" (24 percent).

Recent reviews indicate that among patients under treatment, especially for chronic, asymptomatic conditions such as hypertension, up to 50 percent of patients fail to keep follow-up appointments and 50 to 60 percent fail to take medications regularly [Caldwell et al., 1970; Haynes and Sackett, 1974; Blackwell, 1973; Podell, 1975]. The tendency of physicians to underestimate the frequency and importance of nonadherence makes it a particularly difficult problem.

Nonadherers as described by Blackwell [1973] are:

> those with chronic illnesses requiring long-term maintenance, with suppressive or preventive treatment. The ill-effects of stopping medication may be subtle or remote rather than dramatic or immediate. Children, the elderly and the disadvantaged can cooperate less readily. Patients with hostile feelings toward doctors or those with risk-taking, obsessional, paranoid or hypochondriacal personalities may be unwilling to comply. The patient will be more likely to take medication prescribed by a familiar, well liked physician who believes in the importance of medication and adopts a reassuring attitude to treatment or side effects. Finally, medication is more likely to be taken if

the number of drugs is few, the frequency of taking them is less and the side effects are minimal. Those who are most closely supervised in the hospital or at home are most likely to comply. [Blackwell, 1973]

To these factors should be added poor understanding of the medication regimen [Svarstad, 1974]. It is clear that the problem of poor adherence is a complex one and that the illness, the patient, the physician, the patient–physician relationship, and the medication regimen are all involved.

An attempt to synthesize these multiple factors affecting patient behavior into a systematic framework is the Health Belief Model [Becker and Maiman, 1975]. In this, adherence is conceived to be the result of the interaction of the health motivations of an individual, the perceived value of reducing the threat of the specific illness, and the probability that adherence will reduce this threat. Barriers or obstacles to health care, conflicting motives or priorities, social and cultural values, and triggers or cues to action all influence the final outcome, as do psychological traits of the patient, including defense mechanisms and coping styles. Though of questionable clinical utility, this model does succeed in focusing attention on potentially important factors affecting adherence.

Better knowledge of the predictors of nonadherence is essential if interventions are to be rationally designed and targeted at individuals most likely to benefit from them.

INTERVENTIONS TO IMPROVE ADHERENCE

Hypertension, because it is frequently asymptomatic and because treatment, once begun, is usually of lifelong duration, provides unique challenges to efforts to improve adherence. The reinforcement provided by the relief of symptoms, as with many acute illnesses, is not available. Patients, therefore, must take medications on faith, hoping that doing so will prevent future complications, and must be willing to trade the inconvenience, side effects and costs of treatment for these potential future benefits. Given these circumstances, efforts to improve adherence have focused on increasing the convenience of medical care, on education of the patient and the provider, and on improving the provider–patient relationship. Recently, provision of tangible rewards to patients for adherent behavior has been proposed as an additional approach.

IMPROVING ACCESS TO HEALTH CARE.   Greater convenience of health care services, including shortened waiting times and improved continuity of the relationship with a provider, have been shown to reduce clinic dropout rates significantly [Finnerty, Mattie, and Finnerty, 1973]. Administrative mechanisms to improve the rate of appointment keeping, including postcard and telephone reminders, have also proven successful [Shepard and Moseley, 1976], although the relationship between appointment keeping and medication adherence has not been demonstrated.

Another approach to making health care more convenient has been to provide services at the place of work. One such program reported a 97 percent follow-up rate and an 81 percent control rate for blood pressure after one year [Alderman and Schoenbaum, 1975]. A well-designed randomized trial, however, was unable to demonstrate any difference in either dropout rates or "compliance" when clinics established at industrial work sites were compared with private physicians providing services after hours [Sackett et al., 1975]. The adherence rate (pill counts indicating consumption of 80 percent or more of prescribed medications) in both settings was only 50 percent, and control rates were approximately 20 percent. A more stringent definition of control in the latter study at least partly accounts for these discrepant results.

Thus, convenience may, but does not inevitably, improve adherence. Because "convenience" may have different meanings for different individuals and in different communities, approaches to improving it should be individualized.

Another barrier to access is the cost of treatment. This affects primarily those with no health insurance or insurance that does not adequately cover ambulatory care and medications. Until comprehensive health insurance or prepaid health care is universally available, financial barriers will continue to interfere with the management of hypertension.

PATIENT EDUCATION.   Knowledge of hypertension has been demonstrated to be insufficient to ensure adherence [Sackett et al., 1975; Tagliacozzo and Ima, 1970]. Conditioning factors, such as intervening social circumstances at home or work, may be required to translate knowledge into adherence. Furthermore, education coupled with behavioral strategies may be successful. In one study the augmentation of physician care by a pharmacist, who identified gaps in patient understanding of the disease and the medical regimen and monitored adherence, was able to increase adherence from 25 to 79 percent [McKenney et al., 1973]. Improvements did not persist, however, after the intervention was stopped. In another study involving physicians only, intensive instruction to ensure understanding of regimens, along with encouragement to adhere, was associated with a striking improvement in adherence [Svarstad, 1974].

On balance, evidence suggests that, to be successful, patient education programs should consider patient perceptions, attitudes, values, and social milieux in addition to knowledge per se. Because of well-demonstrated deficiencies in patient memories, frequent reinforcement is a prerequisite [Joyce et al., 1969; Ley and Spelman, 1965; Horwitz, 1976]. Individual instruction by the doctor, nurse, or pharmacist, and small group discussions for patients with hypertension, are both channels requiring further exploration.

In addition to one-on-one or small group interventions, public education through the mass media, including radio, television, newspapers, magazines, and posters in public places, has been employed extensively for a variety of public health problems, most notably smoking, and may be effective in altering health behavior. Witness the recent reports of a decrease in the smoking rate of middle-aged males from 60 to 40 percent.

A study currently in progress under the auspices of Stanford University provides more direct evidence [Curry et al., 1976]. After two years, differences found between three comparable small towns indicate that intense exposure to a mass media campaign is effective in improving health behavior in relation to the cardiovascular risk factors, including hypertension. The long-term effectiveness of such interventions remains to be proven, however.

PROVIDER EDUCATION.   Education of providers both to improve technical competence and to impart attitudes requisite to the successful management of a chronic condition such as hypertension is receiving increased emphasis [National High Blood Pressure Education Program, 1973c]. Specific focus on the adherence problem in tutorial sessions with physicians has been shown to lead to improvement in patients' knowledge of their disease and to increased rates of blood pressure control [Inui, 1973]. Emphasis on factors in the physician–patient interaction that lead to improved understanding of therapeutic regimens and their justification also seems to be effective [Svarstad, 1974].

Existing programs of continuing education for physicians have failed, however, to demonstrate changes in behavior or improved quality of care as a result [Opfell, 1973; Miller, 1967; Williamson, 1965]. Perhaps they focus too much on factual knowledge and not enough on the patient care process.

Another approach has been to educate nurses and other health personnel to assume responsibility for the long-term management of hypertension under the supervision of physicians. Training focuses specifically on the technical and attitudinal skills required to manage hypertension. Experiences to date indicate a high degree of patient acceptance of such personnel and equal or improved quality of care as a result [Sackett et al., 1974; Spitzer et al., 1974; Komaroff et al., 1974; Lewis and Resnik, 1967; Starfield, Sharp, and Mellits, 1971].

Further efforts to improve the ability of the physician to manage chronic diseases such as hypertension are clearly needed. Likewise, expanded use of other personnel may help greatly to extend physicians' services. Educational programs should recognize the shared responsibility of patients and providers in the complex process of managing hypertension successfully.

INCENTIVES FOR ADHERENCE. A promising approach to the adherence problem currently under study is the use of tangible incentives—money, merchandise, or the adjustment of insurance premiums—to reward desired health behaviors. Because, in comparison to other interventions, this requires a relatively small investment of professional time, cost-effectiveness stands to be favorable.

Applications of incentives in industry and commerce are many and have been in use for decades. Monetary rewards to employees based on measures of output, given as bonuses or incentive payments and coupled with information feedback, have led to substantial increases in productivity [Opsahl and Dunnette, 1966; Parsons, 1974]. Incentives in the form of merchandise or services, termed "premiums," to both employees and consumers are widely used—a total of five billion dollars in 1973 [Blood, 1973, 1974]. These are exemplified by gifts offered by banks for opening accounts or by distributors to salesmen for good sales performance. In the life insurance industry, some companies have allowed adjustment of insurance premiums toward standard rates for those policyholders with hypertension who demonstrate consistent reductions in blood pressure [National Heart and Lung Institute, 1974].

Incentives have also been used to encourage desired health and social behaviors in mental hospitals, prisons, and schools [Kazdin, 1975]. Behavioral contracting has proven successful in the management of alcoholism and smoking. Under this approach the patient contracts with a person important to him, generally a spouse or a therapist, to limit his smoking or drinking behavior, in return for which the other person offers reciprocal promises, such as refraining from criticism. Positive and negative consequences, such as increased attention and monetary fines, respectively, are specified in the contract [Pomerleau, Bass, and Crown, 1975].

One of the most extensive applications of the behavioral approach, and the one most closely related to hypertension, has been in the control of obesity [Katz and Zlutnick, 1975; Mann, 1974]. Virtually all previous weight control therapies have been failures since patients either lost no weight or readily regained any they had initially lost [Stunkard and McLaren-Hume, 1959]. Behavior modification in the form of rewarding weight loss or improvements in eating habits or physical activity has been the only approach to obesity that has been demonstrably successful [Stunkard, 1975].

The design of incentives to improve adherence to antihypertensive regimens should take into account certain critical principles. First, behaviors to be rewarded must be clearly spelled out, observable, and under the patient's control. For hypertension these might include appointment keeping, prescription filling, pill taking, and blood pressure control provided that pharmacological resistance and inadequate prescription practices are excluded. The more immediately the incentive relates to the desired behavior, the more effective it is likely to be. Second, the rewards must be perceived as valuable and fair by the participants in relation to the prerequisite behaviors. Finally, the person issuing the rewards should be perceived as caring about the participants. Feedback and praise for performance may well enhance the efficacy of incentives. The rewards themselves might take the form of money, merchandise, or access to sweepstakes giving the participant a chance at a much larger prize.

If such an intervention proved effective, its potential applications would be many. Life insurance companies could offer incentives to policyholders of group or individual policies. Incentives would be particularly attractive because the cost of antihypertensive treatment does not affect the life insurance company, whereas the reduction in the risk of death or disability does.

Health insurers represent another possible user. They can reduce the costs of treating the complications attributable to uncontrolled blood pressure by improving adherence, but, unlike the life insurance companies, they would also pay much of the increased cost of treatment. Because, as shown in chapter 2, treatment of hypertension incurs more costs than it saves, incentives cannot be justified for a health insurer on the basis of cost savings alone. High visibility, public relations, and marketing advantages may more than offset these added costs, however.

Incentives may be most useful to employers and unions concerned about the health and welfare of their work forces. Large groups are usually "experience-rated" with regard to health, life, and disability insurance, meaning that the insurance premium charged is based on the past and projected experience of the group in filing claims. Thus, if the use of incentives makes a group more healthy, the employer or union will benefit. Similarly, absenteeism due to sickness may be decreased and losses due to premature retirement, disability, or death of employees reduced. Possibly more important, incentives can demonstrate to an employee that his employer or union cares about his health and welfare, thereby helping to raise his morale, productivity, and desire to remain with his present employer or union.

IMPACT OF INCOMPLETE ADHERENCE ON THE COST-EFFECTIVENESS OF TREATMENT FOR HYPERTENSION

It has been argued that, because individuals frequently fail to adhere to prescribed therapy, attempts to screen for and treat hypertension in the community may be unwise [Sackett, 1974]. If resources are spent detecting, referring, diagnosing, and initiating treatment only to have a large fraction of patients subsequently fail to continue with treatment, then benefits per dollar spent are severely diluted. The magnitude of the effects of incomplete adherence on the cost-effectiveness of treating known hypertensives is assessed in this section, and analysis of the cost-effectiveness of screening for hypertension in the presence of incomplete ad-herence is presented in chapter 5.

The fundamental question to be answered is this: Does treat-ment that appeared worthwhile under the assumption of full adherence continue to appear so under incomplete adherence, or does it become so expensive per unit of health benefit derived that it becomes an unattractive use of resources? The answer depends upon the proportion of the potential health benefits from treat-ment that is actually received as a function of the rate of ad-herence, and upon the proportion of treatment costs that continues to be consumed by patients dropping out or only partially adhering to prescribed regimens.

METHODS.   To estimate the effects of incomplete adherence on the benefits of medical treatment, a matrix depicting the com-ponents of adherence has been formulated (table 4.1). Param-eters considered include: the average proportion of prescribed pills taken daily; the proportion of days in any specified period of time during which this proportion of the daily prescription was taken; and the proportion of one's life during which this level of treatment was maintained (allowing for dropouts or discontinuous medical care). Based on the product of these proportions, the "fraction of effect," or expected proportion of benefits received relative to full adherence, was estimated.

Three major assumptions underlie the formulation. First, it was assumed that the prescribed regimen is optimal and, if fully adhered to, would successfully reduce the patient's diastolic blood pressure from 110 mm Hg to 90 mm Hg, according to the stepped control schedule (table 2.3). The problems of pharmacological resistance and inadequate prescription practices were thus ex-cluded. Second, it was assumed that there is a linear relationship between the proportion of the daily prescription taken and the resultant benefits and side effects. Actually, there is evidence on both sides of this issue. Some evidence upholds the theory that half the regimen gives *more* than half the benefit (because the first 10 mm Hg reduction in blood pressure yields more benefit than the next 10 mm Hg). Other evidence supports the alternative hypothesis that half the regimen gives *less* than half the benefit (because of threshold effects in dose-response or because irregular drug-taking habits result in detrimental fluctuations in blood pres-sure). Since neither side is much more convincing than the other, the intermediate point of view was adopted. The third assumption

Table 4.1: Adherence matrix.

(1)	(2)	(3)	(4)	(5)	Maximum cost assumption			Minimum cost assumption		
Adherence type	Frequency in treated population	Fraction of dose per day	Fraction of days	Fraction of life	Fraction of effect[a]	Fraction of treatment cost (MD)	Fraction of treatment cost (Drugs)	Fraction of effect[a]	Fraction of treatment cost (MD)	Fraction of treatment cost (Drugs)
1	2/9	1	1	1	1	1	1	1	1	1
2	2/9	1/2	2/3	1	1/3	1	1	1/3	2/3	1/3
3	2/9	1/3	1/2	1	1/6	1	3/4	1/6	1/2	1/6
4	2/9	~0	~0	1/6	~0	1/6	1/6	~0	1/6	1/6
5	1/9	1	1	1 year[b]	~0	1 year	1 year	~0	1 year	1 year
Average					0.33[c]	0.67[d]		0.33[c]	0.42[e]	

[a] Product of columns (3), (4), and (5).

[b] Patient assumed to be under treatment for one year only and then to drop out of medical care.

[c] Weighted average over all adherence types. Applies to benefits and side effects, and to the costs and quality loss associated with morbid events. Equivalent to a fraction of effect of 0.50 among nondropouts (types 1–3).

[d] Based on weighted average of costs over all adherence types, assuming that drugs represent 70% ($140/$200) of treatment costs. Equivalent to 1.00 times treatment cost per nondropout (types 1–3). When converted to dollars, 1/9 of one year's cost must be added (for type 5).

[e] Based on weighted average of costs over all adherence types, assuming that drugs represent 70% ($140/$200) of treatment costs. Equivalent to 0.625 times treatment cost per nondropout (types 1–3). When converted to dollars, 1/9 of one year's cost must be added (for type 5).

was that no benefits accrue to the patient on days he fails to take any pills. The prolonged duration of action of some antihypertensive agents was thus ignored.

Five general types of adherence behavior were identified and assumed to be distributed in the population of known, treated hypertensives as noted under "Frequency" in table 4.1. This distribution is consistent with evidence from a number of hypertension surveys which indicate an early dropout rate (types 4 and 5) of one-third [Wilber and Barrow, 1972; Schoenberger et al., 1972; Harris, 1973][1] and variable adherence among those who continue with treatment (types 1, 2, and 3). The resultant net effective adherence rate is one-half [Wilber and Barrow, 1972; National High Blood Pressure Education Program, 1973e].

Costs of treatment include medications, doctor visits, and required laboratory examinations. In this analysis the upper and lower bounds of these are considered to vary with the level of adherence according to assumptions of "maximum cost" and "minimum cost" (table 4.1). Under the former, incomplete adherers are assumed to continue to use resources at the same rates as full adherers. Medications are purchased but not consumed, and physicians are visited but prescriptions not followed. The average "fraction of cost" absorbed by those who remain in treatment is hence 1.0, and cost-effectiveness is adversely affected. Dropouts from medical care incur no direct costs of treatment. The minimum cost assumption, on the other hand, holds that patients continue to visit physicians as before, but purchase medications only in proportion to consumption. Under these circumstances, the net impact on cost-effectiveness will be smaller because costs are reduced.

RESULTS.   Cost-effectiveness results for treatment under full adherence (tables 2A.4 and 2A.5) serve as a baseline. Comparison of results under full adherence and incomplete adherence for the maximum cost and minimum cost assumptions, by age and initial diastolic blood pressure, appear in tables 4.2 and 4.3 for males and females, respectively; results specific for diastolic blood pressure reductions from 110 mm to 90 mm Hg are dis-

---

1. The dropout rate of one-third is also consistent with independent estimates that about one-half of identified hypertensives remain in treatment [National High Blood Pressure Education Program, 1973e]. If three-quarters of newly identified hypertensives commence therapy [Harris, 1973], then the present situation is in equilibrium if two-thirds of those who commence therapy continue therapy, since $2/3 \times 3/4 = 1/2$.

Table 4.2: Effect of incomplete adherence on the cost-effectiveness[a] of treatment for males.

Age	Diastolic blood pressure (mm Hg)	Full adherence	Incomplete adherence	
			Minimum cost assumption[b]	Maximum cost assumption[b]
20	90	$11,000	$13,900	$21,700
	100	5,500	6,930	10,800
	110	3,270	4,060	6,280
	120	2,130	2,660	4,080
30	90	14,700	19,400	30,400
	100	6,940	8,960	14,100
	110	4,000	5,130	8,040
	120	2,570	3,280	5,140
40	90	19,200	23,000	38,300
	100	9,230	12,100	19,100
	110	5,190	6,670	10,600
	120	3,210	4,180	6,740
50	90	33,900	38,600	68,300
	100	12,800	15,800	25,000
	110	6,870	9,270	14,900
	120	3,920	5,220	8,750
60	90	c	c	c
	100	50,100	87,000	103,100
	110	16,300	19,900	32,100
	120	7,750	11,300	19,200

Results are by age at the time of initiation of treatment and by pretreatment diastolic blood pressure. Assumes: age-varying partial benefit; discounting at 5% per annum; stepped blood pressure control.
[a] Net dollar cost per year of increased quality-adjusted life expectancy.
[b] See table 4.1.
[c] Net effectiveness is negative.

played in figures 4.1 and 4.2. Treatment at 110 mm Hg is emphasized because it includes in its range of 105 to 114 mm Hg the lowest blood pressures advocated for routine treatment by the National High Blood Pressure Education Program [1973b].

Cost-effectiveness for both sexes and at all ages deteriorates under incomplete adherence: the cost per year of increased quality-adjusted life expectancy approximately doubles under the maximum cost assumption and increases by 25 to 30 percent under the minimum cost assumption. Thus, incomplete adherence makes treatment of hypertension a much less attractive use of health care resources, especially if the true state of affairs is closer to the maximum cost assumption.

POLICY IMPLICATIONS. In order to examine the implications of these results for the use of national resources, the aggregate cost-effectiveness of treatment of the United States adult popula-

Table 4.3: Effect of incomplete adherence on the cost-effectiveness[a] of treatment for females.

Age	Diastolic blood pressure (mm Hg)	Full adherence	Incomplete adherence	
			Minimum cost assumption[b]	Maximum cost assumption[b]
20	90	$40,100	$56,500	$80,300
	100	14,700	18,700	29,500
	110	8,490	11,100	17,500
	120	5,260	6,800	10,800
30	90	23,600	32,000	50,600
	100	10,600	13,100	20,800
	110	6,520	8,520	13,600
	120	4,100	5,290	8,510
40	90	19,000	24,200	38,400
	100	9,880	12,700	20,400
	110	5,990	7,810	12,700
	120	3,920	5,130	8,530
50	90	18,600	25,600	40,600
	100	9,290	12,100	19,500
	110	6,000	7,970	13,200
	120	3,840	5,200	8,950
60	90	16,200	21,000	33,300
	100	7,970	10,900	17,500
	110	5,030	6,780	11,300
	120	3,220	4,460	7,780

Results are by age at the time of initiation of treatment and by pretreatment diastolic blood pressure. Assumes: age-varying partial benefit; discounting at 5% per annum; stepped blood pressure control.

[a] Net dollar cost per year of increased quality-adjusted life expectancy.
[b] See table 4.1.

tion was estimated by the method used in chapter 2. If treatment were provided to all persons with diastolic blood pressures of 105 mm Hg or above, the average cost per year of increased quality-adjusted life expectancy would be $10,500 under the maximum cost assumption and $6,400 under the minimum cost assumption, compared to only $4,850 under full adherence. Corresponding figures for treatment of persons with diastolic blood pressures from 95 mm Hg through 104 mm Hg are presented in table 4.4.

Estimated annual national costs of treatment for different treatment cutoff blood pressures and different adherence assumptions are shown in table 4.5. Aggregate treatment costs are lower under incomplete adherence because of dropouts and poor adherers. This is particularly evident under the minimum cost assumption. As indicated by comparison of tables 4.4 and 4.5,

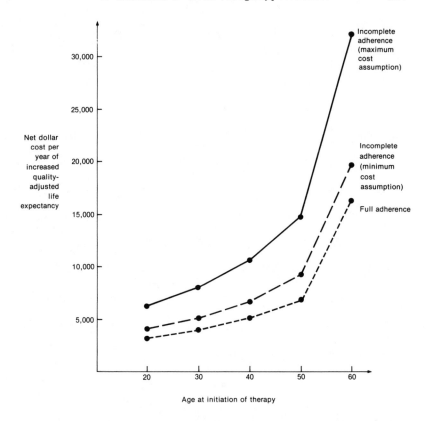

Figure 4.1: Effect of incomplete adherence on the cost-effectiveness of treatment for males, by age at initiation of treatment. Results under the minimum and maximum cost assumptions (table 4.1) are for control of diastolic blood pressure from 110 mm Hg to 90 mm Hg. Assumes: age-varying partial benefit; discounting at 5 percent per annum.

however, cost-effectiveness deteriorates substantially under incomplete adherence despite the decrease in aggregate costs.

A Framework for Evaluating the Cost-Effectiveness of Interventions to Improve Adherence

Since data on the effectiveness and costs of interventions intended to improve adherence rates are so fragmentary, the most that can be done at this time is to make estimates of cost-effectiveness for such interventions and propose an analytical framework within which the policy implications of new data can be assessed as they become available.

One immediate implication of the analytical approach to ad-

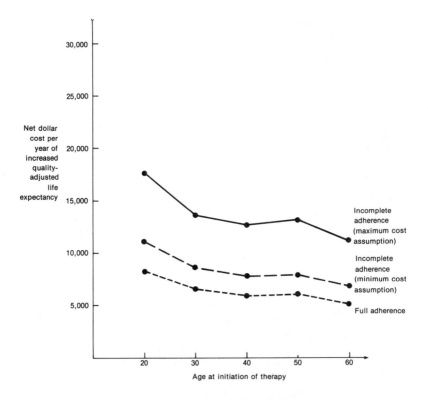

Figure 4.2: Effect of incomplete adherence on the cost-effectiveness of treatment for females, by age at initiation of treatment. Results under the minimum and maximum cost assumptions (table 4.1) are for control of diastolic blood pressure from 110 mm Hg to 90 mm Hg. Assumes: age-varying partial benefit; discounting at 5 percent per annum.

---

herence presented in the previous section is that any intervention that uses additional resources to increase the adherence rate will be more cost-effective if the maximum cost assumption holds than if the minimum cost assumption holds. Under maximum cost, the effective adherence rate for nondropouts is 50 percent while the effective fraction of treatment cost is 100 percent (table 4.1). Thus a program that reduces nonadherence by half would increase the effective adherence rate to 75 percent while increasing costs only by the cost of the proadherence intervention. Under minimum cost, however, the effective fraction of treatment cost is only 62.5 percent, so that a program that would reduce nonadherence by half would also induce cost increases due to increased consumption of medications. The net effect on costs would therefore be an 18.75 percent increase in the cost of treatment, $(100\% - 62.5\%) \times 0.5$, plus the cost of the proadherence

Table 4.4: **Estimated aggregate national cost-effectiveness by severity of hypertension and adherence assumption.**

Pretreatment diastolic blood pressure (mm Hg)	Full adherence	Incomplete adherence	
		Minimum cost	Maximum cost
105 and above	$4,850	$ 6,400	$10,500
95 through 104	9,880	12,500	20,400

Estimates are derived by dividing the average net present-value lifetime treatment costs by the average net increase in quality-adjusted life expectancy.

intervention. Thus, as the minimum cost assumption deals a less severe blow to the cost-effectiveness of treatment, it also renders interventions that increase adherence relatively less cost-effective.[2]

To gain insights into potential cost-effectiveness and, hence, policy implications of interventions to improve adherence, a hypothetical proadherence intervention program was applied to the previously developed model. This program was assumed to involve physicians and nurses in intensive personal interaction with patients, and to increase the cost of treatment by $100 in the first year and $25 per year thereafter. These costs might represent, for example, two hours of additional physician time at $50 per hour in the first year (one-half hour at each of four visits) and one-half hour each year thereafter, or they might represent an equivalent value of nurse time, group or individual instruction in self care, or some combination of these. This would represent

Table 4.5: **Estimated annual national treatment costs (in billions of dollars) by treatment criterion and adherence assumption.**

Pretreatment diastolic blood pressure (mm Hg)	Full adherence	Incomplete adherence	
		Minimum cost	Maximum cost
105 and above	0.9	0.4	0.6
95 and above	2.9	1.2	1.9
90 and above	4.8	2.0	3.2

Estimates are derived by multiplying the number of hypertensive patients potentially treated by $200 times the fraction of cost absorbed under the appropriate adherence assumption (table 4.1).

2. A separate issue entirely is the effect of proadherence interventions on the cost-effectiveness of *screening* for hypertension. In that case the value of such interventions is potentially great under either adherence assumption since pretreatment costs make up a significant portion of the total expenditure on a hypertensive patient. The impact of proadherence interventions on the cost-effectiveness of screening is evaluated separately in the next chapter.

Table 4.6: Impact of an intervention that improves adherence by 50 percent on the cost-effectiveness of treatment for males under the maximum cost assumption.

Age	Diastolic blood pressure (mm Hg)	(1) Cost-effectiveness[a] $\Delta C/\Delta E$	(2) Cost of intervention[b] ΔC_I	(3) Cost-effectiveness with intervention[c] $\dfrac{\Delta C + \Delta E}{\Delta E + \Delta E_I}$	(4) Cost-effectiveness of intervention $\dfrac{\Delta C_I}{\Delta E_I}$
20	90	$21,700	$460	$15,600	$ 9,470
	100	10,800	460	7,780	4,770
	110	6,280	450	4,550	2,850
	120	4,080	440	2,950	1,860
30	90	30,400	440	20,600	12,500
	100	14,100	430	9,800	5,950
	110	8,040	420	5,670	3,440
	120	5,140	410	3,650	2,220
40	90	38,300	400	25,900	17,100
	100	19,100	390	13,100	7,900
	110	10,600	380	7,540	4,490
	120	6,740	370	4,750	2,760
50	90	68,300	350	42,600	29,400
	100	25,000	340	17,800	11,500
	110	14,900	330	10,100	5,870
	120	8,750	320	6,010	3,360
60	90	[d]	290	[d]	[d]
	100	103,100	280	65,600	39,600
	110	32,100	270	22,600	15,100
	120	19,200	260	12,100	6,540

Assumes: age-varying partial benefit; discounting at 5% per annum; stepped blood pressure control.

[a] $\Delta C/\Delta E$ is the net dollar cost per additional quality-adjusted life year as a result of treatment for hypertension under incomplete adherence and the maximum cost assumption.

[b] ΔC_I is the increment in cost due to the proadherence intervention.

[c] ΔE_I is the increment in quality-adjusted life years attributed to improved adherence resulting from the intervention.

[d] Net effectiveness is negative.

approximately a doubling in the personnel costs of treatment assumed in chapter 2.

The impact of this program on the cost-effectiveness of treatment was assessed under the alternative assumptions that it results in a 50 percent or a 20 percent improvement in adherence (that is, from 50 percent to 75 percent or from 50 percent to 60 percent, respectively). The fundamental question addressed is whether or not such a program, expensive as it is, would be justified.

Table 4.7: Impact of an intervention that improves adherence by 50 percent on the cost-effectiveness of treatment for females under the maximum cost assumption.

Age	Diastolic blood pressure (mm Hg)	(1) Cost-effectiveness[a] $\Delta C/\Delta E$	(2) Cost of intervention[b] ΔC_I	(3) Cost-effectiveness with intervention[c] $\dfrac{\Delta C + \Delta E}{\Delta E + \Delta E_I}$	(4) Cost-effectiveness of intervention $\dfrac{\Delta C_I}{\Delta E_I}$
20	90	$80,300	$480	$54,600	$32,800
	100	29,500	480	21,000	12,600
	110	17,500	480	12,100	7,200
	120	10,800	470	7,530	4,470
30	90	50,600	460	32,800	19,600
	100	20,800	460	14,800	9,200
	110	13,600	450	9,370	5,530
	120	8,510	450	6,000	3,490
40	90	38,400	430	27,400	16,300
	100	20,400	420	14,400	8,470
	110	12,700	420	8,890	5,100
	120	8,530	410	5,880	3,300
50	90	40,600	380	26,300	17,200
	100	19,500	380	13,700	7,980
	110	13,200	370	9,120	5,090
	120	8,950	370	6,040	3,120
60	90	33,300	330	23,800	14,200
	100	17,500	320	11,700	7,190
	110	11,300	310	7,790	4,320
	120	7,780	300	5,200	2,630

Assumes: age-varying partial benefit; discounting at 5% per annum; stepped blood pressure control.

[a] $\Delta C/\Delta E$ is the net dollar cost per additional quality-adjusted life year as a result of treatment for hypertension under incomplete adherence and the maximum cost assumption.

[b] ΔC_I is the increment in cost due to the proadherence intervention.

[c] ΔE_I is the increment in quality-adjusted life years attributed to improved adherence resulting from the intervention.

A proadherence program that increases adherence by half significantly improves cost-effectiveness of treatment under both the maximum and minimum cost assumptions although the improvements are more dramatic under the former. Results for the maximum cost assumption are tabulated in tables 4.6 and 4.7 for men and women respectively. For each age and diastolic blood pressure cost-effectiveness is better with the intervention (column 3) than without it (column 1) despite the incremental cost of the intervention (column 2). This occurs because the program is itself more cost-effective than treatment alone (col-

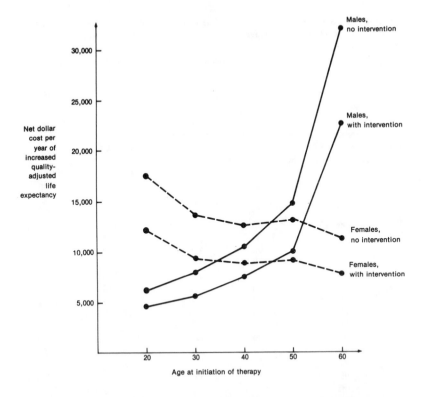

Figure 4.3: Impact of an intervention that improves adherence by 50 percent on the cost-effectiveness of treatment under the maximum cost assumption. Results are for control of diastolic blood pressure from 110 mm Hg to 90 mm Hg. Assumes: age-varying partial benefit; discounting at 5 percent per annum.

umn 4 compared to column 1). Results for control of diastolic blood pressure from 110 to 90 mm Hg are shown graphically in figure 4.3.

A proadherence program that improves adherence by only 20 percent still has a beneficial effect on cost-effectiveness if the maximum cost assumption holds. Under the minimum cost assumption, however, this is no longer true, as shown in tables 4.8 and 4.9 and in figure 4.4. Under these circumstances the intervention itself is less cost-effective than treatment alone and, hence, overall cost-effectiveness deteriorates.

The explanation for differences in results under the two cost assumptions is that under minimum cost, incremental costs are those both of the intervention and of additional medications con-

Table 4.8: Impact of an intervention that improves adherence by 20 percent on the cost-effectiveness of treatment for males under the minimum cost assumption.

Age	Diastolic blood pressure (mm Hg)	(1) Cost-effectiveness[a] $\Delta C/\Delta E$	(2) Cost of intervention[b] ΔC_I	(3) Cost-effectiveness with intervention[c] $\dfrac{\Delta C + \Delta E}{\Delta E + \Delta E_I}$	(4) Cost-effectiveness of intervention $\dfrac{\Delta C_I}{\Delta E_I}$
20	90	$13,900	$420	$15,100	$18,300
	100	6,930	420	7,560	9,140
	110	4,060	410	4,470	5,400
	120	2,660	400	2,880	3,450
30	90	19,400	400	20,300	25,300
	100	8,960	390	9,600	11,600
	110	5,130	390	5,550	6,710
	120	3,280	380	3,570	4,330
40	90	23,000	370	26,800	33,600
	100	12,100	360	12,900	15,600
	110	6,670	350	7,630	9,040
	120	4,180	340	4,630	5,740
50	90	38,600	320	47,700	60,600
	100	15,800	310	18,300	23,200
	110	9,270	300	9,970	12,300
	120	5,220	290	5,990	7,700
60	90	d	260	d	d
	100	87,000	260	71,300	80,700
	110	19,870	250	24,400	32,200
	120	11,340	240	12,200	15,500

Assumes: age-varying partial benefit; discounting at 5% per annum; stepped blood pressure control.

[a] $\Delta C/\Delta E$ is the net dollar cost per additional quality-adjusted life year as a result of treatment for hypertension under incomplete adherence and the minimum cost assumption.

[b] ΔC_I is the increment in cost due to the proadherence intervention.

[c] ΔE_I is the increment in quality-adjusted life years attributed to improved adherence resulting from the intervention.

[d] Net effectiveness is negative.

sumed, while under maximum cost, nonadherers are already purchasing, though not consuming, medications at the rate of full adherers so that the only incremental costs are those of the intervention itself.

Therefore, if reality is closer to the maximum cost situation, efficient use of resources dictates that all categories of patients under treatment should also receive the proadherence intervention. If, however, the minimum cost situation applies, the strength of the intervention becomes much more critical and only selected categories of patients should receive the intervention.

Table 4.9: Impact of an intervention that improves adherence by 20 percent on the cost-effectiveness of treatment for females under the minimum cost assumption.

Age	Diastolic blood pressure (mm Hg)	(1) Cost-effectiveness[a] $\Delta C/\Delta E$	(2) Cost of intervention[b] ΔC_I	(3) Cost-effectiveness with intervention[c] $\dfrac{\Delta C + \Delta E}{\Delta E + \Delta E_I}$	(4) Cost-effectiveness of intervention $\dfrac{\Delta C_I}{\Delta E_I}$
20	90	$56,500	$440	$55,200	$64,300
	100	18,700	440	20,400	24,800
	110	11,100	430	11,800	14,200
	120	6,800	430	7,350	8,900
30	90	32,000	420	32,700	38,800
	100	13,100	420	14,800	18,300
	110	8,520	410	9,170	11,100
	120	5,290	410	5,820	7,150
40	90	24,200	390	26,600	32,540
	100	12,700	390	14,010	17,210
	110	7,810	380	8,630	10,680
	120	5,130	380	5,790	7,290
50	90	25,600	350	26,300	31,450
	100	12,100	350	13,400	16,550
	110	7,970	340	8,870	11,110
	120	5,200	340	5,970	7,690
60	90	21,000	300	23,230	28,800
	100	10,900	290	11,600	14,300
	110	6,780	290	7,600	9,670
	120	4,460	280	5,180	6,820

Assumes: age-varying partial benefit; discounting at 5% per annum; stepped blood pressure control.

[a] $\Delta C/\Delta E$ is the net dollar cost per additional quality-adjusted life year as a result of treatment for hypertension under incomplete adherence and the minimum cost assumption.

[b] ΔC_I is the increment in cost due to the proadherence intervention.

[c] ΔE_I is the increment in quality-adjusted life years attributed to improved adherence resulting from the intervention.

The rule of efficient allocation of resources is that the cost-effectiveness ratio for treatment at the blood pressure cutoff level for treatment should be equal to the marginal cost-effectiveness ratio for the proadherence intervention at the cutoff level for the intervention. Hence, if treatment at a given blood pressure is more cost-effective than the intervention, then resources can be profitably shifted by lowering the cutoff pressure for treatment and raising that for the intervention. Conversely, if the intervention is more cost-effective than treatment at some pressure, then resources can be profitably shifted by raising the cutoff pressure

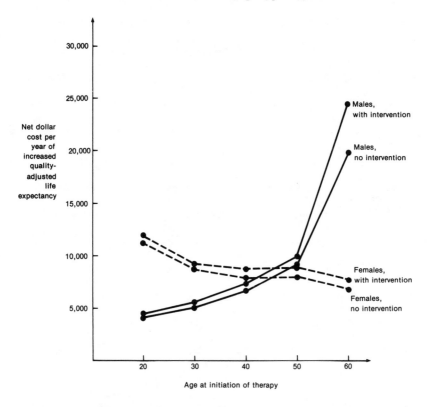

Figure 4.4: Impact of an intervention that improves adherence by 20 percent on the cost-effectiveness of treatment under the minimum cost assumption. Results are for control of diastolic blood pressure from 110 mm Hg to 90 mm Hg. Assumes: age-varying partial benefit; discounting at 5 percent per annum.

for treatment and lowering that for the intervention. Obviously, the cutoff for the intervention cannot be lower than that for treatment. Thus, under the maximum cost assumption, for either a 50 percent or 20 percent improvement in adherence, the best possible solution is, in effect, to set a single cutoff level and offer the intervention to all patients treated. For the minimum cost assumption the same would hold for 50 percent improvement, but for 20 percent improvement the cutoff level for the intervention should be higher than that for treatment.

This optimal allocation principle is illustrated in figures 4.5 and 4.6. Figure 4.5 shows, for males, the cost-effectiveness of treatment alone by age and pretreatment blood pressure under incomplete adherence. Figure 4.6 shows the marginal cost-effectiveness for a proadherence intervention that increases adherence

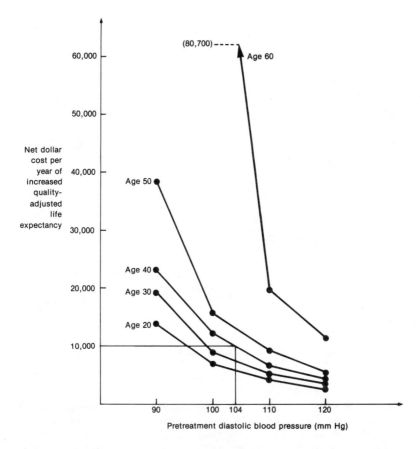

Figure 4.5: Cost-effectiveness of treatment for males under incomplete adherence and the minimum cost assumption, by age and pretreatment blood pressure. Assumes: age-varying partial benefit; discounting at 5 percent per annum; stepped blood pressure control.

by 20 percent. If budgetary restrictions or preferences are such that the policy maker is able or willing to invest only in interventions that cost no more than $10,000 per quality-adjusted year of life saved, then the cutoff level for treatment in 40-year-olds would be 104 mm Hg (figure 4.5), and that for the proadherence intervention would be 109 mm Hg (figure 4.6). Thus it would be efficient to treat 40-year-old men with blood pressures above 104 mm Hg, but to offer proadherence interventions only to those whose blood pressures are above 109 mm Hg.

Up to this point the discussion has assumed that the unit cost and effectiveness of proadherence interventions are the same for all patients. If such is not the case, targeting of the interventions

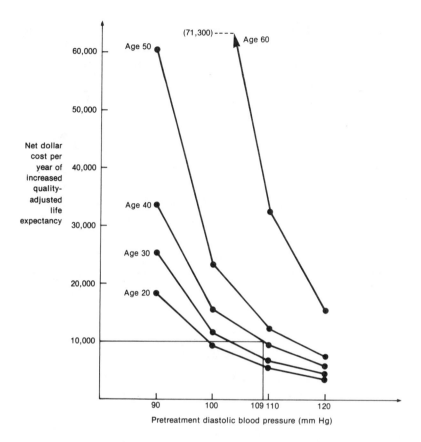

Figure 4.6: Cost-effectiveness of a proadherence intervention that improves adherence by 20 percent under the minimum cost assumption. Results are for males, by age and pretreatment diastolic blood pressure. Assumes: age-varying partial benefit; discounting at 5 percent per annum; stepped blood pressure control.

at subsets of patients for whom they are most cost-effective should be considered. Contrary to many widely advocated strategies, this does not necessarily mean targeting at the worst adherers. Instead the object should be to target at categories of patients for whom the expected increase in adherence, multiplied by the benefit per unit change in adherence, is greatest relative to the cost of the intervention. This may mean targeting at patients who are most likely to respond, even if they are already reasonably adherent: better to increase the proportion of adherent patients from 70 percent to 90 percent than from 20 percent to 25 percent. The criterion also suggests the value of targeting at those who would receive the greatest benefit were they to adhere to therapy, as determined by age, sex, and blood pressure level parameters, and, possibly, the coexistence of other cardiovascular risk factors such as smoking and high serum cholesterol.

While the physician who knows his patients well may be able to predict with some accuracy their individual propensities to adhere, evidence to date indicates few if any population characteristics that are reliable predictors of adherence. Therefore, while the potential is great, it remains for future research to determine how to improve the efficiency of antihypertensive care by targeting proadherence interventions at responsive groups.

This analysis of the cost-effectiveness of interventions to improve adherence to antihypertensive treatment is intended to be suggestive rather than definitive. While the potential cost-effectiveness of increasing adherence is great, actual cost-effectiveness remains to be demonstrated. Certainly, much more must be learned before the wisdom of a massive public policy initiative to improve adherence can be supported with confidence.

Conclusions

The cost-effectiveness of treatment for hypertension depends not only on its efficacy in reducing blood pressure and cardiovascular risk but also, very importantly, on the degree to which patients remain under medical care and adhere to prescribed regimens. Provider as well as patient behaviors bear critically upon this problem. Using evidence currently available, this analysis indicates marked deterioration of the cost-effectiveness of treatment under incomplete adherence; particularly for mild hypertension, treatment becomes a relatively unattractive use of health care resources.

Interventions to improve adherence can, potentially, greatly increase the efficiency of hypertension management. Public, patient, and provider education, emphasis on the provider–patient relationship, better access to medical care, and tangible incentives offered for desired health behaviors, used alone or in combinations, all are avenues warranting serious exploration. The potential for targeting at specific subpopulations, and the need for reinforcement over the lifetimes of hypertensive patients, must also be considered.

Implementation of proadherence interventions will depend critically on the organizational structures of the health care settings involved. Methods feasible and appropriate in a hospital out-patient department, health maintenance organization, or neighborhood health center may be different from those for the private physician. Because 85 percent of patients receive their primary care from private physicians [Harris, 1973], particular efforts need to be focused in this area.

Better understanding of factors underlying health behaviors and the design and evaluation of interventions to affect these favorably are major challenges for the future. Such efforts should be given very high research priority, since they bear heavily on the ultimate efficacy and cost-effectiveness of hypertension control programs.

5. Detecting Hypertension

From 19 to 59 percent of United States hypertensives are unaware of their condition [Wilber and Barrow, 1972; Schoenberger et al., 1972; National High Blood Pressure Education Program, 1973e]; this presents a problem of major dimensions. Lack of contact with medical care providers, failure to measure blood pressure during encounters, inadequate communication between provider and patient, and denial of the condition's existence by the patient are all responsible. Several alternative approaches to this problem have been proposed. Public education aimed at motivating people to seek regular medical care, provider education to encourage early detection and treatment of hypertension, and public screening programs all have their advocates and critics. Public and provider education have received increased attention under the impetus of the National High Blood Pressure Education Program. Our major focus, however, is upon screening for hypertension, because of the vigorous debate that this approach has generated, and because of the numerous screening programs that have been mounted or are being planned [American Heart Association, 1974].

The fundamental policy issue is whether screening for hypertension is a cost-effective use of health care resources. Two competing considerations are involved. On the one hand, screening itself is a relatively inexpensive way to identify large numbers of hypertensive individuals. On the other hand, its ultimate effectiveness depends upon the likelihood that an individual will reach a provider of care, that the provider will administer effective antihypertensive therapy, and that the patient will continue in care and adhere to that therapy.

Public and Provider Education

Under the aegis of the National High Blood Pressure Program and the American Heart Association considerable efforts have been made in recent years to increase public awareness of the importance of high blood pressure as a health problem [National High Blood Pressure Education Program, 1973d; American Heart Association, 1974]. Mass media campaigns through television, radio, the press, and distribution of posters and written materials have been conducted on national, state, and local levels. National High Blood Pressure Months each year since 1974 have served to highlight these efforts. School health programs designed to impress upon young people the importance of prevention are being explored. To date, however, the impact of these wide-ranging programs is unknown.

On a local level, in a controlled trial involving three comparable but independent communities in California, an intensive mass media campaign has shown encouraging effects on preventive health behavior with respect to a variety of cardiovascular risk factors, including hypertension [Haskell et al., 1974; Curry et al., 1976]. Further evaluation of the effectiveness and cost of public health education is clearly required before major new resources are devoted to this approach [Green, 1974].

Even under conditions of enhanced public awareness of the importance of hypertension, the provider is a vital link in the process of identifying individuals at risk and initiating treatment. Blood pressures must be taken in the course of encounters, the results and meaning of these conveyed to the patient, and appropriate referral, diagnostic, and treatment measures begun. The importance of provider behavior is recognized in the detailed recommendations for performance characteristics, learning objectives, and evaluation approaches for provider education programs prepared by the National High Blood Pressure Education Program [1975, 1973c]. That problems exist is clearly indicated by the frequency with which many providers fail to measure blood pressures during encounters [Frohlich et al., 1971] or fail to respond to identification of risk factors at screening [Aronow, Allen, and De Cristofaro, 1975].

Solutions being attempted are many. Programs of continuing education for physicians are being offered, though, unfortunately, the effects of these on physician behavior have been difficult to ascertain [Opfell, 1973; Miller, 1967; Williamson, 1965]. Family practice and primary care residency programs have burgeoned to train physicians whose major objectives are to encourage sound preventive health practices and to care for common or chronic illnesses. Finally, training of nurses and other personnel to assume major responsibilities for the management of chronic illnesses is being explored. Though all of these approaches show promise, it is too early to estimate the impact they will have on the early detection and treatment of hypertension.

Screening

Screening is the direct approach to increasing awareness and initiating the patient management process. It may be defined as active efforts on the part of health care providers to diagnose a condition or disease in individuals who, whether asymptomatic or symptomatic, have not themselves sought medical care for the condition or the symptoms related to it. Operationally, screening may take place either as a part of an ongoing health care process or in the form of categorical outreach programs aimed at the detection of one or more conditions in a target population.

The rationale for screening in general [McKeown, 1968; Thorner, 1970; Whitby, 1974] and for hypertension screening in particular [American Heart Association, 1974; Sackett, 1974] has been vigorously debated within the medical profession and, recently, has begun to emerge as an issue of public interest as well. While a fair consensus exists regarding the criteria that should ideally guide the decision to screen, implementation of these has been inconsistent, and public policy remains very much a matter of controversy.

The cost-effectiveness analysis presented here extends the analyses of chapters 2 and 4 to include screening. Community-wide screening, strategies of targeting screening by race and age, and screening by the provider as part of an ongoing health care process are all considered.

RATIONALE FOR SCREENING

The primary purpose of screening for hypertension is to detect its presence in an asymptomatic stage before irreparable damage has occurred [McKeown, 1968; Whitby, 1974]. Early detection of hypertension is valued to the extent that early treatment either prevents or delays the development of symptomatic cardiovascular disease, including stroke, heart attack, and congestive heart failure. Additional benefit derives if early treatment also reduces the net expected lifetime health care costs of the population screened. For hypertension, however, the latter is not the case since, in aggregate, the costs of treatment exceed the expected savings from the treatment of cardiovascular diseases prevented (see chapter 2). Reduction of the probabilities of very high-cost outcomes for some individuals is possible, however, and, for these, screening may be considered to be a form of insurance, mitigating the effects of such outcomes. (Such "insurance" would have value, however, only if individuals or third-party payers are risk-averse [Raiffa, 1968].)

Other rationales for screening might apply even if treatment were not effective. Relief of anxiety may accrue to those found not to have the condition, for example, to those who have a family history of hypertension and fear its consequences. Conversely, the possibility exists that anxiety will be created needlessly in those who are erroneously identified as hypertensives or who cannot be treated effectively. Reduction of uncertainty about one's future health status, thus permitting sounder future planning in such personal matters as management of financial resources, insurance, pensions, retirement, and family responsibilities, may also be of value.

Indirect benefits may accrue as well. For some individuals, screening may provide an entry point into comprehensive health care. For the health care system, it may serve as a tracer for the quality of health care in a community and, as such, may be used as a signal that improvements are needed. Finally, advocates of health care, particularly in urban areas, support blood pressure screening to gain political support for their causes in the neighborhoods they represent.

CRITERIA FOR COST-EFFECTIVE SCREENING

To assess in a qualitative way whether screening for hypertension is an attractive use of health resources, a series of questions has been formulated and addressed. These were derived in part from the literature [McKeown, 1968; Whitby, 1974] and in part from considerations that arose during the present analysis. The ultimate decision will involve tradeoffs between the strengths and weaknesses of a proposed program as assessed against these questions. The ensuing quantitative analysis attempts to incorporate explicitly the tradeoffs identified here.

Is the condition serious enough to justify the effort? Evidence is conclusive that elevated blood pressure is a major cause of death and disability [Kannel and Gordon, 1974]. Few conditions are as important in terms of mortality and morbidity.

Is the prevalence of the condition high enough to justify screening? The National Health Examination Survey of 1960–1962 indicates that 17 percent of the United States adult population have blood pressures above 160/95 mm Hg [National Center for Health Statistics, 1964a]. In selected ethnic groups and geographic regions the percentage is even higher. Compared with most conditions, this is an extraordinarily high prevalence.

Is an inexpensive, benign, and accurate screening test available? Blood pressure measurement with a sphygmomanometer is inexpensive, requiring only a few minutes of a health professional's time and minimal capital expense. There is virtually no associated pain or discomfort. Accuracy is, however, a problem, both because of technical considerations (equipment errors or biases) and the known fluctuations of true blood pressure within individuals in response to daily activities and stresses. Surveys indicate that 32 to 54 percent of persons found to have elevated blood pressures at primary screening ultimately do not prove to have hypertension [Wilber and Barrow, 1972; Oberman et al., 1974; Alderman and Schoenbaum, 1975; Charman, 1974; Finnerty, Shaw, and Himmelsbach, 1973]. This is obviously a significant problem. However, because low test specificity (that is, the probability of a negative finding when the condition is absent) is most important when the prevalence of the condition being sought is low,[1] it is not fatal to screening for hypertension, though it does affect cost-effectiveness unfavorably.

What are the consequences of a false positive test? False positive screening test results may have several adverse consequences, including anxiety needlessly aroused and the costs and risks of unnecessary diagnostic procedures and treatment. Careful secondary screening can substantially reduce the number of false positives, but its additional costs must be considered.

---

1. The ratio of true positives to false positives is equal to [(Sensitivity) × (Prevalence)]/[(1 − Specificity) × (1 − Prevalence)]. If the prevalence is very small, the specificity will have to be close to unity to avoid a ratio that is almost as small as the prevalence.

How likely is it that an individual found to have the condition will reach a treatment source? Failure of referral from screening programs to health care providers can be a major problem. The referral rate achieved depends greatly on the particular setting in which screening occurs, the commitment of the involved personnel to patient follow-up, and the relationship between the screening program and sources of medical care. Too often the objective of community screening programs is merely to screen, perhaps because screening is visible and thus may be a vehicle for political purposes. For hypertension, the problem of referral is especially difficult, because the patient is usually asymptomatic and because treatment does not result in any immediate or dramatic benefit.

Is an effective treatment available, and, if so, what are its costs and risks? This is a most important question for any screening program whose rationale is prescriptive, as opposed to investigative or epidemiological. McKeown says regarding prescriptive screening that "there is then a presumptive undertaking, not merely that abnormality will be identified if it is present, but that those affected will derive benefit from subsequent treatment or care" [1968]. For hypertension, the case for the effectiveness of treatment is persuasive for moderate and severe elevations (diastolic blood pressures greater than 105 mm Hg), though the magnitude of benefits remains uncertain. For patients with milder hypertension, who make up nearly 80 percent of the total hypertensive population, greater uncertainty exists. Likewise, as demonstrated in chapter 2, the case for cost-effectiveness is strong for some classes of patients (for example, young men and all patients with diastolic pressures above 115 mm Hg), but tenuous for others (older men and those with diastolic pressures under 105 mm Hg). Side effects of therapy also must be considered. Mild, and frequently subjective, side effects are very real and very common. More serious side effects are rare but devastating when they occur. Both detract from the positive benefits of treatment. Net effectiveness of treatment in different categories of patients remains a major issue in judging the value of hypertension screening programs.

Is the effectiveness of treatment significantly greater if the condition is detected in its asymptomatic stage? Assuming that blood pressure reduction is effective in preventing death and cardiovascular disease, it is reasonable to assume that the benefits of treating asymptomatic hypertension are greater than those of waiting until the symptoms of heart disease or stroke present themselves. Definitive evidence, however, must await the results of controlled trials involving both asymptomatic and symptomatic hypertensive patients. Because the Veterans Administration Cooperative Study [1972] was composed predominantly of patients with preexisting evidence of cardiovascular disease, it alone cannot provide the answer. The Hypertension Detection and Follow-Up Program and United States Public Health Service studies which are currently in progress may.

Does the health care system have the capacity to treat the newly found cases? The burden imposed upon available health care facilities by the identification of patients requiring diagnostic services and long-term treatment may be severe. If successful, public screening for hypertension could result in more than 10 percent of the population being referred. There is doubt whether the capacity of health care facilities and providers, in some parts of the country at least, could accommodate such a demand unless it were spread over a period of time sufficient to permit redistribution and expansion of existing resources. Results of too rapid a referral rate could be a refusal or inability of health care providers to accept referred hypertensive patients, or restriction of services provided for treatment of other health problems. To the extent that excess capacity in the system exists, however, the relatively predictable treatment demands of a condition such as hypertension may increase efficiency by smoothing demand and hence be less costly than would be the case if new capacity were required.

How likely is it that the patient will adhere to prescribed long-term treatment? As discussed in chapter 4, this may be the single most important question in evaluating the net effectiveness and cost-effectiveness of screening for hypertension. Poor adherence has been clearly shown to be a significant problem with hypertensive patients. Unless patient education or other interventions prove effective in improving adherence, this problem alone may be sufficient to dictate against widespread blood pressure screening. Without adherence there is no therapy, and without therapy there can be no benefit.

Is public screening necessary? Even if the answers to all of the above questions were favorable to screening, this would imply only that early detection is worth pursuing, not that categorical public screening is indicated. McKeown [1968] argues that public responsibility for screening may derive from any of three sources. To these we add a fourth.

First, in communicable disease, public intervention is often justified because the health risk imposed by an individual carrying the disease extends beyond the individual himself. Where contagion is possible, individual incentives to be screened and treated may be insufficient relative to the social value of such actions. Society's remedy is often to provide screening and treatment publicly. This is the rationale for public management of tuberculosis and venereal disease, but it does not apply to hypertension.

Second, public screening may be justified if there is research value to be derived. This is, in effect, a public good that no individual would have the incentive to provide; hence public intervention is required. Except for studies such as the Hypertension Detection and Follow-Up Program, however, the primary purpose of most hypertension screening programs has not been research.

The justification for public screening for hypertension lies, if anywhere, in McKeown's third category, prescriptive screening, that is, intervention for the patient's own good. Public provision of prescriptive screening may be justified on at least two bases. First, people may, and in fact do, lack information about the value of screening for asymptomatic conditions such as hypertension and therefore fail to seek care on their own. Education is one possible remedy, but direct screening may be more cost-effective. Second, some argue that it is a public responsibility to ensure that people do, in fact, receive care for conditions that benefit from early treatment, even if they do not actively seek care on their own despite having the requisite information and access to care. This argument is tenuous, at best, from the point of view of possible infringement on individual rights. Were it the only one, community screening for hypertension would be difficult to justify.

A fourth possible justification of screening lies in the financial basis under which public or private health insurance plans operate. When individuals are insured, they have diminished incentives to minimize their own health care costs since the net cost to each individual is spread throughout the premium structure. Thus, an individual who fails to take action to minimize his health care costs is, in effect, passing on the costs to others who share the premium. Collective action may be indicated in such circumstances to protect the group against the adverse, though not necessarily malicious, behaviors of its members. In conditions for which the savings from early treatment outweigh the treatment costs, this would be a major rationale for public screening. For hypertension, because of the net financial cost imposed by its treatment, the basis for public screening must lie in the health benefits it provides.

PRIVATE AND PUBLIC APPROACHES

Both private screening as an intrinsic part of the health care process and categorical public screening have been advocated and employed in the United States. Despite the fact that a substantial majority of the population has contact with the health care system on a regular basis [National Center for Health Statistics, 1973a], nearly half of all hypertensives identified by screening programs are unaware of their condition [Wilber and Barrow, 1972; Schoenberger et al., 1972; National High Blood Pressure Education Program, 1973e]. This discrepancy suggests either that blood pressure is not measured when health care is sought for other purposes, or that the results are not communicated to, or remembered by, the patient. Possible remedies include increased efforts by individual providers to detect and treat or refer hypertensives, or public screening programs to supplement regular health care channels.

PRIVATE SCREENING.   Between 67 and 84 percent of patients visit physicians yearly and more than 90 percent do so every five years [National Center for Health Statistics, 1973a]. Hence, if its ultimate potential were realized, private screening would reach the vast majority of the population. If, in addition, blood pressure were measured routinely by dentists, oculists, optometrists, and pharmacists, an even larger proportion of the population would be reached.

That this potential has not been realized reflects both the nature of the health care system and the attitudes of providers toward hypertension. A large proportion of health care is delivered in response to a medical "crisis" or specific patient complaints. In this context, blood pressure measurement is frequently omitted [Brook and Appel, 1973; Frohlich et al. 1971]. Increased emphasis on continuing comprehensive health care, and promulgation of standards and guidelines through such bodies as peer review organizations, may alleviate this problem.

One advantage of screening as a routine part of health care is that it requires only a few minutes of a nurse's or health aide's time and hence involves little additional expenditure of resources. Furthermore, because the majority of the public feels that the physician is a "very reliable source of information" [Harris, 1973], positive results are more likely to be believed. Moreover, because treatment is provided either directly by the screener or by a colleague to whom the patient is referred, problems of referral are minimized.

A major limitation of private screening is that those individuals who are isolated from the health care system for geographic, economic, educational, or attitudinal reasons will be missed. If these could be identified, however, they might be suitable targets for outreach screening.

PUBLIC SCREENING. Public screening has the potential of reaching large numbers of people at moderate cost. Support has derived from diverse sources including community and service organizations, professional and medical associations, city, county, and state governments, health care institutions including hospitals and neighborhood health centers, academic and research organizations, insurance companies, and drug companies.

Screening programs have varied widely with respect to screening methods employed, characteristics of target populations, arrangements for rescreening or referral, and funding mechanisms. Screening has been performed at places of employment and schools, at home by door-to-door canvass, and at temporary locations such as mobile vans, shopping centers, churches, and meetings or conventions. Some of the most significant community outreach programs will be described briefly.

The Connecticut High Blood Pressure Program of the Connecticut Heart Association and the City of New York Department of Health Program have demonstrated their abilities to reach large numbers of individuals in a variety of community settings. Shortcomings have included their failure to provide for secondary screening, difficulties in ensuring effective referral to medical care facilities, and their tendencies to attract patients already aware of and, frequently, already under treatment for hypertension. This latter fact was particularly well demonstrated in a study in Atlanta in which fewer than 20 percent of hypertensives identified were unaware of their condition [Wilber and Barrow, 1972]. Apparently, those who already knew that they had hypertension were attracted disproportionately to the program.

The Hypertension Detection and Follow-Up Program, a federally funded collaborative trial involving fourteen centers, is another model. Screening was performed, in large part, by door-to-door canvassing with subsequent rescreening and treatment provided at local health care settings. Very high rates of ascertainment and of subsequent follow-up were achieved, but at a very high cost. Though tolerable for a program with research objectives, it is doubtful whether such costs could be borne by ongoing service programs.

Finnerty and his colleagues, in Washington, D.C., have demonstrated some of the pitfalls and prerequisites of successful public screening [Finnerty, Shaw, and Himmelsbach, 1973]. By screening in supermarkets they were able to reach 61 percent of an adult, urban, and predominantly black target population and identify 24 percent of these as having blood pressures greater than 140/90 mm Hg. Initially, however, only 50 percent of those referred for rescreening kept their appointments. By scheduling appointments within forty-eight hours this rate was increased to 95 percent, indicating the importance of reinforcing the message conveyed by the first knowledge of elevated blood pressure at the earliest possible time. Despite all efforts, however, only 30 percent of those originally identified as having elevated blood pressures were ultimately available for treatment, the others being categorized as either false positives or dropouts. The relatively low blood pressure level chosen as the cutoff for the primary screen undoubtedly contributed to this low retention rate.

Screening at industrial sites and other places of employment has been evaluated in a number of studies [Schoenberger et al., 1972; Alderman and Schoenbaum, 1975; Charman, 1974; Sackett et al., 1975]. Advantages of such programs include their convenience for the target population in terms of both their location and hours of operation. Problems related to the use of company time to screen employees and the need for confidentiality of results have been successfully circumvented by obtaining union and management endorsements. The question of whether industrial populations are appropriate targets for screening programs because of hiring practices that tend to exclude people with elevated blood pressures is another issue, however, which may adversely affect the cost-effectiveness of such programs.

Each type of public screening program has intrinsic advantages and disadvantages. Effectiveness depends importantly on the demographic characteristics of the population being screened and on the closeness of the relationship between the screening program and community medical resources. Screening targeted at high-risk, high-prevalence populations such as blacks is likely to be more cost-effective than community-wide screening, as is demonstrated in the subsequent analysis.

To the extent that such programs reach individuals who do not otherwise use health care facilities, they are of particular value. There is no definite information available on this point, but it is likely that the majority of those who appear for screening already have a high level of concern about their health in general or about hypertension in particular. A further advantage of public screening is its high degree of visibility, and its consequent ability to increase community awareness of the importance of hypertension as a health problem.

Balanced against these positive attributes are the problems such programs face in maintaining quality control of blood pressure measurement techniques, thus limiting the adverse consequences of false positives, and in ensuring adequate provision for rescreening and referral.

Cost-Effectiveness Analysis of Screening for Hypertension

The cost-effectiveness of screening for hypertension is affected by the benefits and costs of treatment, by medication side effects that mitigate benefits achieved, and, especially, by incomplete patient adherence and attrition between screening and the initiation of treatment. This quantitative analysis combines these considerations and permits conclusions about whether hypertension screening, either community-wide or targeted at particular groups, is an efficient use of health resources.

DATA SOURCES AND ASSUMPTIONS

Because of the limitations of available data and the need to supplement them with subjective estimates, the conclusions reached should not be viewed as universal or definitive, but rather as logical consequences of the data and assumptions that were adopted. Individual decision makers can apply their own data and estimates of uncertain parameters to the analytic framework to reach conclusions applicable to their own situations.

Data on population-based distributions of diastolic blood pressures by age and sex were obtained from the National Health Examination Survey (NHES) of 1960–1962 [National Center for Health Statistics, 1964a]. Since the NHES measurements were also based on the average of several repeated blood pressure readings in individuals, the residual false positive rate was assumed to be comparable to that in the Framingham Heart Study [Kannel and Gordon, 1974], which provided the basis for the benefit calculations in this analysis. Prevalences were adjusted to account for the fact that today a larger fraction of a screened population sample would be under treatment than in 1960–1962. Data from the National High Blood Pressure Education Program [1973e] imply that one in eight hypertensives is under control. In 1960–1962, because therapy was infrequently administered to all but severe hypertensives, the proportion under control at that time was assumed to be zero. Data from the study by Wilber and Barrow [1972] were used to estimate the rate at which prior awareness increases with higher blood pressure.

The data relating to costs and benefits of treatment by age, sex, and pretreatment blood pressure were developed in chapters 2 and 4. Four alternative assumptions regarding adherence were used: (1) full adherence; (2) incomplete adherence with the maximum cost assumption (table 4.1), in which nonadherers who remain in treatment continue to absorb treatment resources at the same rate as adherers; (3) incomplete adherence with maximum cost as ameliorated by a hypothetical follow-up intervention that improves adherence by 50 percent (chapter 4); and (4) incomplete adherence with the minimum cost assumption (table 4.1), in which nonadherers absorb only a proportionate fraction of medication costs.

Assumptions made regarding the costs of screening, measurement errors, and attrition prior to treatment are as follows:

• Primary screening was assumed to cost $6 per individual, including publicity, record keeping and other ancillary requirements. This estimate is an average based on the experiences of a number of screening programs [American Heart Association, 1974; Oberman et al., 1974]. Because screening costs are overwhelmed by those of diagnostic evaluation and treatment, lower values would not significantly affect the results of the analysis.
• False negatives at primary screening were assumed to be

negligible, but false positives were assumed to compose one-third of all detected diastolic blood pressures above 95 mm Hg (that is, a predictive value positive, or true-positive rate, of 0.67). Typical estimates of predictive value positive derived from actual programs range as low as 0.50, but center around 0.67 [Wilber and Barrow, 1972; Finnerty, Shaw, and Himmelsbach, 1973].

• Secondary screening, involving repeated blood pressure readings, was assumed to eliminate all false positives in excess of those that underlie the NHES and Framingham data and to cost $15 per patient. This cost assumes one additional visit to a physician solely for rescreening prior to the visit at which treatment is initiated.

• Finally, it was assumed that only half of those with positive primary screenings proceed to secondary screening [Wilber and Barrow, 1972], and that three-quarters of those confirmed positive ultimately commence treatment [Harris, 1973]. This assumes that secondary screening occurs in a physician's office. Otherwise, the referral rate to secondary screening might be higher (for example, if secondary screening were done in the same place as primary screening), but the rate of initiation of treatment might be proportionately lower.

THE MEASURE OF COST-EFFECTIVENESS OF SCREENING

The efficiency of screening is measured as the expected dollar cost per unit of health benefit received, expressed in terms of increased quality-adjusted life expectancy. This cost-effectiveness ratio, R, is defined by:

$$R = \frac{\bar{C}}{\bar{E}} = \frac{C_S + \sum_{i \in T} (p_i/p_{TP})p_{SS}C_{SS} + \sum_{i \in T} p_{Rx}C_i}{\sum_{i \in T} p_i p_{Rx}E_i}, \tag{5.1}$$

where:

$\bar{C}$ = expected net cost per individual screened;

$\bar{E}$ = expected net benefit per individual screened;

C_S = expected unit cost of primary screening (= $6);

C_{SS} = expected unit cost of secondary screening (= $15);

p_{SS} = probability that a patient referred to secondary screening will in fact receive it (= 0.5);

p_{TP} = probability that a screened hypertensive is a true positive (= 0.67);

p_{Rx} = probability that treatment is actually administered if the patient is in a category to be treated (= 0.75 × 0.5 = 0.375);

i = index for patient category (by age, sex, and diastolic blood pressure);

p_i = prevalence of patient category i in screened population;

C_i = net present-value lifetime cost of treatment for patient category i under the relevant adherence assumption;

E_i = increase in present-value quality-adjusted life expectancy for patient category i under the relevant adherence assumption;

T = set of categories i for whom treatment is indicated.

This ratio provides a measure of the efficiency of a hypertension screening program that can be compared to analogous measures for other programs for hypertension or other health problems.

The numerator of the cost-effectiveness ratio is the expected dollar cost per individual screened, $\overline{C}$. This is the sum of (1) the cost of the primary screen itself, (2) the cost of secondary screening for those who reach that stage, and (3) the expected treatment and follow-up cost for each category of patient treated. The cost of the primary screen is represented as C_S (equation 5.1). The expected cost of secondary screening per individual screened is the unit cost of secondary screening, C_{SS}, multiplied by the proportion of the screened population who reach secondary screening. This proportion is the sum of the prevalence (p_i) of all categories of patients for whom treatment is to be provided (T), inflated by a factor accounting for false positives at primary screening (p_{TP}), and deflated by a factor accounting for attrition in the referral process (p_{SS}). The expected treatment and follow-up cost per individual screened is the sum, over all categories of treated patients, of the products of prevalence (p_i) and expected net, category-specific, treatment and follow-up costs (C_i), deflated by a factor accounting for failure to initiate treatment following secondary screening (p_{Rx}). It is implicitly assumed that if treatment is not indicated, no further follow-up costs are incurred for that patient.

The denominator of the cost-effectiveness ratio is the expected health benefit per individual screened, $\overline{E}$. This is simply the sum

of the category-specific health benefits (E_i), expressed in terms
of increases in quality-adjusted life expectancy, weighted by the
respective category prevalences (p_i), and deflated by the fraction
of these for whom treatment is actually initiated (p_{Rx}).

EFFECT OF TREATMENT CRITERIA ON THE COST-EFFECTIVENESS OF A SCREENING PROGRAM

The choice of criteria for initiating treatment for hypertension
has a major effect on the overall cost-effectiveness of screening.
If it were decided to treat all hypertensives with confirmed
diastolic pressures of 105 mm Hg or above, as recommended by
the National High Blood Pressure Education Program [1973b],
then the set of treated categories of patients, T, would include
the blood pressure groups 110 mm Hg (105–114 mm Hg) and
120 mm Hg (115 mm Hg and over). If the cutoff level were 95
mm Hg, the set T would then include, in addition, all patients in
the blood pressure group 100 mm Hg (95–104 mm Hg). Another criterion might be to treat all hypertensives for whom the
ratio of cost to effectiveness for treatment alone (chapter 2), or
treatment including adjustment for nonadherence (chapter 4), is
under some arbitrary level, say $10,000, noting that including
categories for which this ratio, C_i/E_i, is low has a favorable
effect on the overall cost-effectiveness ratio R for screening
(equation 5.1). Under each of these criteria, the cost-effectiveness
ratio for screening would then be computed by including the
appropriate patient categories in the summations in the numerator
and denominator.

It is important to recognize that there is a tradeoff between
screening and treatment implicit in the cost-effectiveness criterion. If screening were free (C_s and $C_{ss} = 0$), then the most
efficient use of resources obviously would be to screen everyone
and treat only the patients with the lowest ratio of cost to effectiveness. If, on the other hand, screening were costly, it would be
more efficient to divert resources from screening to treatment by
relaxing the criterion for treatment (that is, by lowering the
cutoff blood pressure levels and expanding the treatment set, T).
In this case, it would be better to settle for less health benefit per
dollar spent on treatment than to squander resources on screening
until the very most "cost-effective" patients are found. The
optimal criterion for treatment, therefore, would be to select the
set, T, of treated categories so that the ratio, R, in equation 5.1

is minimized. This implies that each dollar spent is yielding the maximum possible benefit and, therefore, that resources are being allocated between screening and treatment in the most efficient possible manner. This optimization is accomplished by first ranking patient categories by their respective treatment efficiencies (C_i/E_i), as calculated in chapters 2 and 4, and then adding them sequentially into the formula for R in order of increasing C_i/E_i until the ratio reaches its minimum. This will occur when the individual cost-effectiveness ratio of the last category included in the treatment set is just equal to the overall cost-effectiveness ratio, R. Beyond that point, including additional categories (for example, lower blood pressures) will increase the ratio and reduce the efficiency of the screening program.

The treatment criterion that optimizes the efficiency of screening was computed under each adherence assumption, and the optimal efficiency of screening thereby derived. An example of this calculation is given in the appendix to this chapter.

ESTIMATED EFFICIENCY OF COMMUNITY-WIDE SCREENING

Cost-effectiveness calculations for screening for hypertension in a representative population subsample of the United States under different treatment criteria and adherence assumptions are given in table 5.1. It is assumed that the individuals screened are representative of the target population.

If all patients with diastolic blood pressures of 105 mm Hg and above are treated, the cost associated with the saving of one quality-adjusted year of life by means of community-wide screening is estimated to be $7,000 if full adherence holds. This increases to about $12,400 for incomplete adherence under the minimum cost assumption, and to about $16,700 for incomplete adherence under the maximum cost assumption (that is, if treatment resources are used at the same rate as under full adherence). An intervention that improves adherence by 50 percent (from 50 to 75 percent) under the latter assumption would result in significant savings, improving the cost-effectiveness to $12,400 in this example.

If treatment is provided for all patients with diastolic pressures of 95 mm Hg and above, the cost of providing an added quality-adjusted year of life by means of this program increases to $8,600 with full adherence, to $12,900 and $19,200 with incomplete adherence under minimum cost and maximum cost, respectively,

Table 5.1: Cost-effectiveness[a] of community-wide screening for hypertension, by treatment criterion and adherence assumption.

Treatment criterion	Full adherence	Minimum cost adherence assumption[b]	Maximum cost adherence assumption[c]	Maximum cost adherence assumption with intervention[d]
Treat diastolic blood pressures $\geqslant$ 105 mm Hg	$7,000	$12,400	$16,700	$12,400
Treat diastolic blood pressures $\geqslant$ 95 mm Hg	8,600	12,900	19,200	13,700
Treat if $C_i/E_i <$ $10,000	8,300	11,400	21,000	9,900
Optimal tradeoff between screening and treatment[e]	6,600	11,400	15,500	9,900

[a] Net dollar cost per year of increased quality-adjusted life expectancy.
[b] Assumes that nonadherers absorb only minimal treatment costs.
[c] Assumes that nonadherers continue to absorb full treatment costs.
[d] Assumes that an intervention reduces nonadherence by half, at a cost of $100 in the first year of treatment and $25 per year thereafter.
[e] See appendix to this chapter.

and to $13,700 in the latter case if the proadherence intervention is added. If an arbitrary cutoff level of $10,000 for the cost-effectiveness ratio for treatment is used, the cost-effectiveness of screening ranges from $8,300 to $21,000.

Finally, if resources are divided between treatment and screening according to the optimization procedure described above, then the cost per year of life saved is only about $6,600 in the best case (full adherence), $11,400 and $15,500 under the two cost assumptions for incomplete adherence, and $9,900 with the proadherence intervention.

Thus, regardless of the criterion chosen for treatment, incomplete adherence to medical regimens seriously compromises the attractiveness of using health care dollars to screen for hypertension. Allocation of resources to efforts to improve adherence in known hypertensives may well prove more efficient than widespread screening without such efforts. This can be seen by comparing the cost-effectiveness of screening with and without the proadherence intervention (table 5.1).

Optimal criteria for treatment by age, sex, and pretreatment blood pressure suggested by the analysis deserve emphasis. Under full adherence, treatment is indicated for "mild" hypertensives (95–104 mm Hg) only for men under age 25. For pretreatment diastolic pressures of 105 mm Hg or above, however, treatment should be provided for all age and sex categories except for men over age 55 in whom it is indicated only if pressures exceed 115 mm Hg. Under incomplete adherence with minimum cost, however, the optimal criteria for treatment are relaxed somewhat in the direction of treating lower blood pressures because more screening resources are needed to find an adherent patient. In this case, it is efficient to treat "mild" hypertension (95–104 mm Hg) in men up to age 35, and in women over age 55.

On a national level, the total cost of primary and secondary screening for hypertension would be "only" about $1.1 billion. This estimate is based on $6 per adult in the United States population and $15 per person given secondary screening, assuming referral of all persons with measured diastolic blood pressures above 95 mm Hg, and 50 percent attrition in the referral process. To this cost, of course, must be added the lifetime costs of treatment and follow-up. To serve as a guide for policy decisions, these total costs should be measured relative to health benefits derived (table 5.1). Thus, while screening per se may not be costly, it may not be cost-effective either, when the obstacles to effective blood pressure control are recognized.

Targeted Screening by Race and Age

A question most relevant to policy determinations is whether or not the efficiency of a screening program for hypertension can be improved by targeting it at selected populations. Even if it is not cost-effective to conduct community-wide programs, screening of selected populations might improve efficiency significantly.

Such target populations might be selected according to any of a number of criteria: (1) high prevalence of elevated blood pressures, (2) high potential benefit of treatment, (3) attractive cost-effectiveness of treatment, or (4) high likelihood of adherence. The latter may be the most appealing of all, since adherence has been shown to be such a major factor in determining the cost-effectiveness of screening (table 5.1). Limited ability to identify characteristics of a population that are predictive of adherence compromises its usefulness at present, however.

Targeting according to age is another potentially attractive strategy, given the wide variability in the cost-effectiveness of treatment, especially among men. The advantages of screening younger men in terms of the cost-effectiveness of treatment are erased, however, by disadvantages resulting from the low prevalence of elevated blood pressures in this group. Age groups for which treatment is most cost-effective are also those for which case-finding is most expensive. For women, both prevalence and cost-effectiveness of treatment are favorable to screening older groups, but the returns are insufficient to justify the higher unit costs associated with locating and screening such a limited population. By all age criteria, the reduction in cost per quality-adjusted year of life saved was found to be no more than $100 to $200.

Far more encouraging than targeting by age is targeting by race. As seen in table 5.2, the frequency distribution of diastolic blood pressures is significantly higher for blacks than for whites. (The same is true of systolic pressures.) The difference of means is about 5 mm Hg for both men and women. These differences in the prevalence of diastolic blood pressures of 95 mm Hg and above, and in the severity of hypertension when present, suggest that screening in black populations might be more cost-effective than screening general populations.

Cost-effectiveness estimates were computed using the blood pressure distributions for black adults alone [National Center for Health Statistics, 1964b], and are shown in table 5.3. Under full adherence, the cost-effectiveness ratio for screening blacks with optimal treatment criteria is $5,300 compared with $6,600 in

Table 5.2: Percent distribution of diastolic blood pressures for United States adults, by race and sex.[a]

Diastolic pressures above (mm Hg)	Males		Females	
	White	Black	White	Black
95	9.0%	22.7%	8.3%	21.5%
100	4.7	10.4	4.7	14.1
105	2.6	6.9	2.5	10.2
110	1.2	4.8	1.3	6.6
115	0.7	2.3	0.9	5.0
120	0.4	1.2	0.4	2.7
125	0.2	0.7	0.2	1.9

[a] From the National Center for Health Statistics [1964b].

Table 5.3: Cost-effectiveness[a] of targeted screening of black adults, by treatment criterion and adherence assumption.

Treatment criterion	Full adherence	Minimum cost adherence assumption[b]	Maximum cost adherence assumption[c]	Maximum cost adherence assumption with intervention[d]
Treat diastolic blood pressures $\geq$ 105 mm Hg	$6,100	$ 9,000	$13,100	$ 8,600
Treat diastolic blood pressures $\geq$ 95 mm Hg	8,600	11,500	17,800	12,000
Treat if $C_i/E_i <$ $10,000	7,500	8,800	12,900	8,400
Optimal tradeoff between screening and treatment[e]	5,300	8,600	12,200	7,900

[a] Net dollar cost per year of increased quality-adjusted life expectancy.
[b] Assumes that nonadherers absorb only minimal treatment costs.
[c] Assumes that nonadherers continue to absorb full treatment costs.
[d] Assumes that an intervention reduces nonadherence by half, at a cost of $100 in the first year of treatment and $25 per year thereafter.
[e] See appendix to this chapter.

general populations. Under other adherence assumptions, the ratio is similarly reduced.

It can be concluded that targeted screening by race improves the efficiency of resource use by 15 to 25 percent (table 5.5). High prevalence and high potential benefits, together with the fact that proportionately fewer blacks are under effective medical care, combine to make screening of black populations an extremely promising avenue to explore.

PRIVATE SCREENING BY THE PROVIDER

An alternative to public outreach screening is to rely upon providers to screen their own patients. Advantages, as stated previously, include reduced cost, reduced attrition between screening and rescreening, and improved likelihood that treatment will be initiated once the diagnosis of hypertension is established. Following screening, incomplete adherence remains the only major obstacle to effective blood pressure control. Such a strategy takes advantage of the fact that most Americans have visited a physician within the last three years, most typically as a "regular source" of care [Harris, 1973]. A disadvantage, however, is the fact that the significant minority of individuals who do not have a regular source of health care will not be screened. Therefore, while it may be more efficient, dollar for dollar, to concentrate the screening effort in existing provider settings, the total magnitude of the benefits achievable might be less than with really effective public screening. This would be a particular problem if high-prevalence, high-potential-benefit groups such as blacks were missed disproportionately.

Estimates of the potential cost-effectiveness of private screening were made, assuming that the probability of referral (p_{ss} in equation 5.1) and the probability of initiation of treatment if indicated (p_{Rx} in equation 5.1) are both one (table 5.4). As shown in table 5.5, the results obtained are 15 to 25 percent better than those obtained by community-wide public screening, and approximately equal to those for public screening targeted by race. Results would be even further improved if the reduced costs of private screening were taken into account.

Table 5.4: Cost-effectiveness[a] of private screening for hypertension, by treatment criterion and adherence assumption.

Treatment criterion	Full adherence	Minimum cost adherence assumption[b]	Maximum cost adherence assumption[c]	Maximum cost adherence assumption with intervention[d]
Treat diastolic blood pressures $\geq$ 105 mm Hg	$5,800	$ 9,000	$13,200	$10,400
Treat diastolic blood pressures $\geq$ 95 mm Hg	8,200	11,600	17,800	13,000
Treat if $C_i/E_i <$ $10,000	7,700	8,600	12,800	8,300
Optimal tradeoff between screening and treatment[e]	5,200	8,400	12,000	7,800

[a] Net dollar cost per year of increased quality-adjusted life expectancy.

[b] Assumes that nonadherers absorb only minimal treatment costs.

[c] Assumes that nonadherers continue to absorb full treatment costs.

[d] Assumes that an intervention reduces nonadherence by half, at a cost of $100 in the first year of treatment and $25 per year thereafter.

[e] See appendix to this chapter.

Table 5.5: Cost-effectiveness summary for hypertension screening.[a]

Adherence	Public screening community-wide	Targeted screening of black adults	Private screening by the provider
Full	$ 6,600	$ 5,300	$ 5,200
Incomplete			
Minimum cost	11,400	8,600	8,400
Maximum cost	15,500	12,200	12,000
Maximum cost with intervention to improve adherence	9,900	7,900	7,800

[a] Net dollar cost per year of increased quality-adjusted life expectancy. Assumes that treatment criteria by age, sex, and blood pressure level optimize cost-effectiveness.

Conclusions and Policy Implications

Based on this analysis, public outreach screening for hypertension on a community-wide basis is not as cost-effective as might be hoped for a preventive health program. Problems of inadequate referral to treatment, unsatisfactory follow-up by providers, and, especially, incomplete adherence to treatment regimens are the fundamental reasons for this result. The cost-effectiveness of community-wide screening would be improved by 30 percent or more, however, if even moderately costly and effective interventions were applied to improve adherence.

The criterion for initiating treatment subsequent to screening is also an important determinant of cost-effectiveness. Relatively high cutoff levels tend to improve efficiency, especially if applied in an age-specific fashion.

Targeted screening in black communities appears to be more cost-effective than community-wide screening due to the higher prevalence of hypertension and its greater severity among blacks. The underlying analysis assumed, however, that adherence is no more of a problem in black than in white populations, but no strong evidence is available that either refutes or supports this assumption.

Screening by providers of health care is likely to be more cost-effective than outreach screening because attrition in referral is minimized. Generalization of this approach, however, would require considerable changes in the attitudes and practices of providers. Changes in medical education and residency training programs are promising approaches to that end. Another

possible approach, given the wide prevalence of fiscal intermediaries in the financing of medical care, is to use financial
incentives to reward providers for effective control of hypertension in their patients or, conversely, to withhold reimbursement
when control is inadequate.

These conclusions suggest that a rational policy might be to
combine public screening in selected populations (black, low
access to care) with efforts to improve provider performance in
the management of hypertension. The merit of these recommendations depends upon our ability to locate, screen, and bring into
treatment selected target populations at a reasonable cost, and
with reasonable adherence, and to provide appropriate education
or professional or financial incentives to providers.

Appendix to Chapter 5

The problem is to find the set, T, of categories of patients to be treated that minimizes the cost-effectiveness ratio for screening (equation 5.1). Substituting the parameter values given in the definitions following equation 5.1, and dividing both numerator and denominator by p_{Rx}, the ratio becomes:

$$R = \frac{(8/3)C_S + \sum_{i\varepsilon T} p_i(2C_{SS} + C_i)}{\sum_{i\varepsilon T} p_iE_i}. \qquad (5A.1)$$

The present example is for the case of full adherence and for screening of the United States adult population, aged 18–64.

The expected costs, benefits, and ratios for treatment alone for the various patient categories by sex, age, and blood pressure, are shown in tables 4.2 and 4.3. The estimated prevalences are those derived from data from the National Center for Health Statistics [1964a] as described in the text.

If no patients are treated, the numerator of R consists only of $(8/3)C_S = \$16$, and the denominator is zero—obviously it is infinitely inefficient to screen if nobody is to be treated. The ratio can be improved by introducing treated categories into the summations in both numerator and denominator.

First we introduce the category of the highest efficiency rank, which happens to be 20-year-old (18–24) males with diastolic blood pressures in the category 120 mm Hg (115 mm Hg and over). However, the prevalence (p_i) of this group is essentially zero, so that we move on to the next group which is 30-year-old (25–34) males with diastolic blood pressures of 120 mm Hg (115 mm Hg and over). For this group we find that $p_i = .0004$, $C_i = 3,411$, and $\Delta E_i = 1.33$. Now the numerator of R is equal to $16 + .0004[(2)(15) + 3,411] = 17.3764$, and the denominator of R is equal to $(.0004)(1.33) = .000532$. The ratio R now stands at \$32,655 per quality-adjusted year of life. This can be improved by treating more categories of patients. As shown in table 5A.1, categories of patients are included in the treatment set through the category of rank 17, at which point $R = \$6,624$ per quality-adjusted year of life. Treating the next category, however, slightly *increases R*. This means that rather than use resources to treat those patients, screening should be continued to seek patients in the other 17 categories. At the margin, of course, not too much would be lost if the eighteenth or nineteenth category of patients were treated. If treatment were given too far beyond the optimal cutoff, however, the efficiency of the program would suffer.

Table 5A.1: Calculation of the cutoff for treatment in optimizing the cost-effectiveness of screening.

Category[a]	Rank	(C_i/E_i)[b]	Cumulative C/E[c]
20M120	1	\$2,126	[d]
30M120	2	2,565	\$32,665
40M120	3	3,210	21,275
60F120	4	3,216	15,359
20M110	5	3,266	15,359[d]
50F120	6	3,843	11,333
40F120	7	3,915	10,413
50M120	8	3,916	9,027
30M110	9	3,995	8,003
30F120	10	4,098	8,003[d]
60F110	11	5,033	7,374
40M110	12	5,188	6,930
20F120	13	5,256	6,930[d]
20M100	14	5,501	6,739
40F110	15	5,992	6,678
50F110	16	6,002	6,626
30F110	17	6,520	6,624 (optimum)
50M110	18	6,865	6,655
30M100	19	6,935	6,698

This example applies to the general United States adult population, and assumes full adherence.

[a] Age-sex-pretreatment diastolic blood pressure (mm Hg).

[b] Category-specific net cost per year of increased quality-adjusted life expectancy.

[c] Including all patient categories for treatment up through this category.

[d] Prevalence of this category is approximately zero.

6. Allocating Resources to Manage Hypertension in a Community

Despite the increasing resources being devoted to the detection and treatment of hypertension, little if any systematic analysis has been done to help policy makers allocate resources efficiently among the various stages in the process from detection to ultimate control. Often the tendency in hypertension programs is to concentrate available funds on screening, and to rely on individuals to seek and continue their own care [Borhani, 1975]. Perhaps, however, while some fraction of available resources may be well spent in finding new cases, a major fraction of those resources might be more productive if shifted to the provision of referral and follow-up services to increase the probability that a hypertensive individual will ultimately be controlled. On the other hand, perhaps the most efficient use of resources is to screen widely, at relatively low cost, accepting the fact that most of those screened will fail to have their blood pressures controlled, rather than to invest in expensive programs (for example, patient education, improving access to health care) to improve adherence to therapy. The question is: given a limited budget, what is the best way to divide it among the several categories of intervention in order to maximize the number of hypertensives brought under control?

This chapter addresses the problem of resource allocation by developing a simple model of the stages involved in the detection and treatment of hypertension. Using data from the literature where available, supplemented by subjective cost and effectiveness estimates where data are not available, tentative conclusions about optimal resource allocation can be derived. The very

Note: The authors of this chapter are Albert L. Nichols, Milton C. Weinstein, and William B. Stason.

166

structure of the model may also provide insights for the decision maker.

A Multistage Model of the Process of Managing Hypertension

The management of hypertension may be viewed as a dynamic process as shown in figure 6.1. It begins with efforts designed to attract people to screening, and ends with adequate control of blood pressure through continued treatment. Interventions, including screening, referral, diagnosis, treatment, and follow-up,[1] are designed to increase the rates of flow of hypertensives along the track to ultimate control (left to right), decreasing the residual dropouts to the several uncontrolled states. The objective is to allocate resources among interventions at the several stages so as to maximize the number of hypertensives achieving the final state of control.[2]

In figure 6.1, eight stages are identified, labeled S_1 through S_8. At each stage, subjects may either continue to the next stage, or they may exit. The probability that a subject will progress from stage S_i to stage S_{i+1} is denoted by p_i, and the probability of exit is $1 - p_i$. The cost per patient at each stage (C_i) includes the basic cost of processing an individual at that stage (for example, screening at S_2, initial treatment at S_6, ongoing treatment at S_7), as well as the costs of any interventions designed to increase the flow rate to the next stage (for example, referral to secondary screening at S_3, or patient education to reduce the dropout rate at S_6 and to improve adherence to medication at S_7). The eight stages in the model are as follows:

Stage 1: *Target population.* The target population may be defined according to its composition with regard to age, sex, race, occupation, and any other characteristics predictive of the prevalence of hypertension or the effectiveness of any of the interventions. It is assumed that all persons start at this stage initially. The probability that a member of the target population is screened is p_1. This may be affected by a number of interventions

---

1. The term "follow-up" is used as shorthand for the wide range of interventions intended to encourage continuation of care and adherence to medical therapy.

2. It is assumed throughout that there is a health benefit deriving from the control of hypertension. Questions as to the magnitude of this benefit are dealt with in chapter 2 but are not essential to the present analysis.

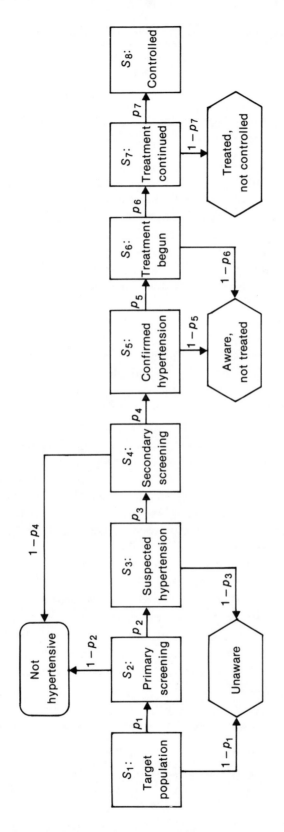

Figure 6.1: A multistage model of the process of managing hypertension.

including public education, efforts to encourage a wide spectrum of health care providers to screen in their practices, or outreach screening programs. The costs per individual in the target population at this stage, C_1, include the costs of these interventions, as well as any overhead costs of providing screening for the population. In a door-to-door screening program, for example, the per capita costs of enumeration and making contact with residents would be included in C_1.

Stage 2: *Primary screening.* Primary screening is defined as the initial measurement (or sequence of measurements) of blood pressure. The probability, p_2, of moving from stage 2 to stage 3 is the probability that a screened individual has a measured blood pressure level above the specified cutoff level. It is determined by the prevalence of hypertension and by the false-positive rate of the screening test (assuming that there are no false negatives). Specifically, p_2 is the prevalence of uncontrolled hypertension in the screened population ($p_2 \times p_4$), divided by the proportion of those screened positive who are truly hypertensive (p_4). The unit cost at this stage, C_2, includes the cost of the actual blood pressure measurement plus any unit costs of administration and record keeping.

Stage 3: *Suspected hypertension.* To reach this stage, an individual must have been screened and found to have an elevated blood pressure. The costs at this stage, C_3, include costs associated with arranging for referral and any educational efforts designed to increase the probability, p_3, that the individual reaches secondary screening. These efforts might range from a verbal recommendation that the individual see his physician, to making an appointment with a physician for the patient, to repeated phone or mail reminders or even home visits.

Stage 4: *Secondary screening.* To confirm the diagnosis of hypertension, repeated measurements of blood pressure are usually necessary. This can be done at a special screening site or at a source of health care. Each alternative has implications for cost and for subsequent progress of treatment. The transition rate p_4 is the probability that the preliminary finding of hypertension is confirmed. Most hypertension screening programs have found high false-positive rates, with as many as half of the suspected hypertensives being eliminated at secondary screening. The unit cost C_4 includes the cost of the blood pressure measurements and any administrative or record-keeping costs.

Stage 5: *Confirmed hypertension.* An individual is confirmed to be hypertensive if an elevated blood pressure is found at secondary screening. The costs at this stage, C_5, are for those interventions intended to increase the probability that the individual will enter care and receive treatment. These may include referral to care, if secondary screening is done at a remote site, and may also include efforts to increase the probability that the individual's source of medical care will initiate treatment. Improved access to health care, patient and professional education, and allocation of resources to the medical sites to which hypertensives are referred, are examples of such efforts. Thus, p_5 is the probability that the confirmed hypertensive reaches a source of care and that treatment is initiated.

Stage 6: *Treatment begun.* This stage includes confirmed hypertensives who begin treatment. Costs here, C_6, include the initial examination by the physician, diagnostic tests ordered, medications for six months, and any follow-up efforts made to ensure continued care. The latter may include patient education, reminders to attend scheduled appointments, and measures taken to improve access to care and to increase the convenience of care. Since many patients drop out of hypertension programs very quickly, the probability of continuing care, p_6, is often low in the absence of such interventions.

Stage 7: *Treatment continued.* Patients who continue treatment for at least six months fall into this category. The problem at this stage becomes one of ensuring adherence to prescribed regimens. Costs at this stage, C_7, are those of lifetime treatment (medications, periodic laboratory examinations, and physician visits) as well as efforts aimed at increasing adherence. The probability that a patient who remains in care has his blood pressure brought under control, p_7, depends on the responsiveness of his blood pressure to prescribed medicines and, even more importantly, on his faithfulness in taking them.

Stage 8: *Controlled blood pressure.* The patient who reaches this stage is a "success." The objective is to divide resources among the interventions at the seven previous stages in such a way as to maximize the chances of reaching this final stage.

A Simple Four-Stage Example

Before the analytic model is developed in its entirety, it is instructive to look at a simplified, hypothetical numerical example that highlights the factors that are important in determining optimal resource allocation among the various interventions. By experimenting with this simple example, it is possible to begin to develop an intuitive feel for the relative importance of, say, screening as opposed to follow-up (that is, proadherence interventions) in maximizing the number of hypertensives controlled under a given budget.

The example (figure 6.2) consists of a four-stage version of the full model. The program starts with a pool of potential candidates for screening. Of those screened, 10 percent are found to have blood pressures at levels determined to justify treatment. It is assumed that the screening procedure is perfectly accurate so that those 10 percent can be classified as "confirmed hypertensives." Of the latter, half are assumed to enter treatment (a simplifying assumption to highlight the tradeoff between screening and follow-up, without complicating the model with intermediate interventions). Of those who enter treatment, it is assumed that in the absence of further intervention 50 percent adhere to therapy and have their blood pressures controlled.

Given this model, the resource allocation problem is as follows. A budget of $1,000,000 is available. Screening (including multiple blood pressure measurements, record keeping, and so on) costs $20 per person. Treatment costs $3,000 per person over the lifetime of the patient. If treatment is made more convenient and an enhanced follow-up program is provided, however, adherence can be increased from 50 percent to 70 percent. Such a service would increase the per-patient cost of treatment by 20 percent, to $3,600. As under the maximum cost assumption of chapter 4, nonadherers are assumed to consume as many resources as adherers.

The question is: under this budget and these assumptions, how should resources optimally be allocated among screening, treatment, and follow-up? Should the maximum possible number of people who can be guaranteed treatment be screened, or should fewer people be screened so that enhanced follow-up can be provided to some or all of those treated? The objective, of course, is to get the most people under blood pressure control subject to the budgetary constraint. In this example, there are two prime alternatives for the optimal allocation. These are (1) to screen that number of people for whom treatment can be guaranteed under the budget, and (2) to screen only that number of people

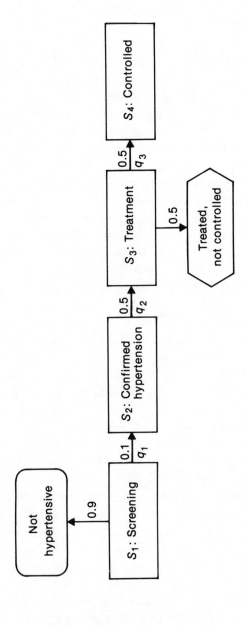

Figure 6.2: Hypothetical four-stage example of resource allocation among hypertensive screening, treatment, and follow-up.

that can be guaranteed both treatment *and* enhanced follow-up.[3] Is it obvious which strategy is optimal?

It is a straightforward matter to compute the expected number of people controlled under each strategy. These computations are shown in table 6.1. Under the "maximum screening" strategy, 5,882 people are screened, but only 147 hypertensives are controlled. Under the "treatment and enhanced follow-up" strategy, only 5,000 can be screened under the budget limitation, but 175 hypertensives are controlled, for a net gain of 19 percent.

Consider the factors that lead to this result. First, note that screening is a relatively cheap way to increase one of the probabilities of passing from one stage to the next (q_1). Provision of screening for $20 with a 0.1 probability of hypertension results in a cost of $2 per percentage point increase in the probability of passing from the first stage to the second stage. Next note that "enhanced follow-up" is a relatively expensive way to increase another transition probability (q_3). Follow-up adds a cost of $600 per patient in treatment and yields an increase of 0.2 ($0.7 - 0.5$) in the final transition probability, for a cost of $30 per percentage point increase in probability. Despite the much greater cost of enhanced follow-up for a given yield of patients to the next stage, the treatment and enhanced follow-up strategy

Table 6.1: Comparison of alternative resource allocation strategies in the hypothetical example.

Number entering stage	Action	Cost per person	Total cost of action	Probability of moving to next stage
Maximum screening strategy				
5,882	screened	$ 20	$118,000	0.10
588	referred	0	0	.50
294	treated	3,000	882,000	.50
147	controlled		$1,000,000	
Treatment and enhanced follow-up strategy				
5,000	screened	20	$100,000	0.10
500	referred	0	0	.50
250	treated and followed up	3,600	900,000	.70
175	controlled		$1,000,000	

3. Because of the linearity of the costs and probabilities, any intermediate strategy (for example, one in which a fraction of those treated are given follow-up) must be dominated by one extreme or the other.

still results in a larger number of controlled hypertensives within a limited budget than the strategy in which a larger number of hypertensives are detected and treated only. Explanation of this apparent paradox lies in the greater efficiency attained when resources are allocated to the later stages of the process (for example, follow-up) than to the initial stages (for example, screening).

The first reason behind this result is that resources applied at an early stage are applied to a larger pool of individuals, many of whom will not make their way through to later stages, while resources applied at later stages are translated directly into controlled hypertensives. A second, and related, reason for preferring intervention at the later stages is that an intervention at the first stage triggers costs at all subsequent stages, especially diagnosis and treatment costs subsequent to screening, for those who reach those stages, while intervention at the last stage triggers no additional costs other than those of the follow-up intervention itself. For both of these reasons, screening may be a much more expensive vehicle for increasing the overall rate of blood pressure control in a community.

The Formal Model

The considerations developed above may be incorporated into a simple, formal model of the resource allocation decision problem, the objectives of which are three: (1) to give qualitative insights into the factors that determine optimal resource allocation, especially between earlier and later stages of the management process, (2) to permit general quantitative policy conclusions to be drawn based on data from the literature regarding costs and yields of interventions, and (3) to provide an analytical framework in which decision makers at the community level can incorporate their own assessments of costs and yields for their programs and thereby derive resource allocations specific to their situations. (Those wishing to proceed directly to the interpretation of results derived from the model are referred to page 180.)

FORMULATION OF THE MODEL

The formal model is as follows. Define F_i ($i = 1, \ldots, 8$) as the probability that a member of the target population reaches stage S_i (figure 6.1). Since an individual must progress through all preceding stages in order to reach S_i, F_i represents the product of the probabilities at each step. Thus, $F_2 = p_1$, $F_3 = p_1 \times p_2$, and so forth. In general:

$$F_i = \prod_{j=1}^{i-1} p_j \qquad (i = 2, \ldots, 8)$$

and

$$F_1 = 1 \qquad (i = 1) .$$

The success rate, or overall effectiveness, of the program is then F_8, or $p_1 \times p_2 \times p_3 \times p_4 \times p_5 \times p_6 \times p_7$.

Implicit in this formulation are two assumptions. First, those who do not achieve blood pressure control are assumed to receive no benefit. (Partial adherence is, however, taken into account if p_7 is interpreted as the average level of adherence in the treated group, as defined in chapter 4, table 4.1.) Second, the transition probabilities achieved are assumed to apply uniformly to all "hypertensives," so that the total health benefits obtained are proportional to the number of hypertensives controlled.

On the cost side, the unit cost at each stage is C_i, and the probability, p_i, is related to the cost through a cost function g_i, so that

$$C_i = g_i(p_i).$$

Assuming that there is a positive and increasing cost associated with achieving marginal increases in the probabilities (mathematically, that the first and second derivatives of the cost function are everywhere greater than zero), a typical cost function might appear as in figure 6.3. The function illustrated has the property that as the transition probability approaches its limit of 1.0, it becomes increasingly expensive to raise it further. For stages where the transition probability and unit cost are fixed, the L-shaped cost function pictured in figure 6.4 would apply. A possibly more realistic assumption than either of these is illustrated by figure 6.5. This formulation posits a base transition probability, p_i^*, associated with a base cost, C_i^*, with improvements in p_i being achievable at an increase in cost above the base level. For example, if $i = 7$, p_i^* is the probability that blood pressure is controlled, given that treatment has been continued for six months and no patient education or proadherence intervention beyond routine treatment is given. Thus, C_7^* is the basic cost of treatment. Increases in p_7 above p_7^* could be achieved if

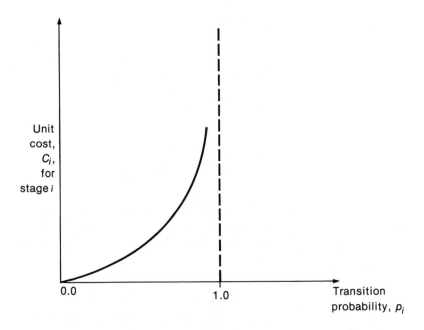

Figure 6.3: Typical cost function relating the unit cost at a given stage to the associated transition probability. This formulation assumes a positive, increasing marginal cost of raising the transition probability.

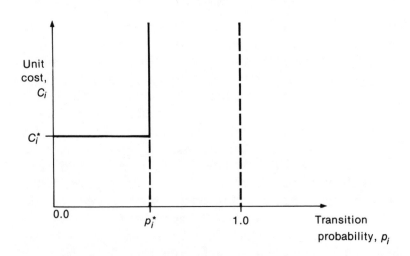

Figure 6.4: Special case cost function where the cost and transition rate are fixed. In this formulation, the unit cost is fixed at C_i^* and the transition probability is fixed at p_i^*. No interventions to increase the transition probability are possible.

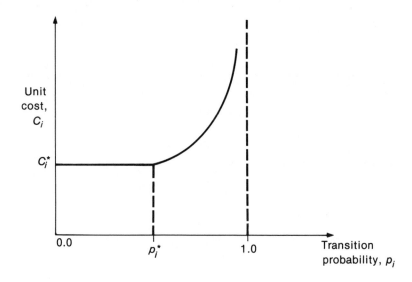

Figure 6.5: Typical cost function where interventions may increase the transition probability above a base level. In this formulation, the "base" transition probability is p_i^*, with a unit cost of C_i^* in the absence of interventions to increase the transition probability. Increases above p_i^* are possible, but at an increasing cost.

the cost were increased above C_7^* to pay for improved access, patient education, or other proadherence measures.

Finally, let A_i denote the per capita cost from the ith stage on to the end of the process. Thus $A_7 = F_7 C_7$, since the only costs remaining at that stage are the costs for the final stage, and a fraction, F_7, of the target population reaches that stage. Similarly, $A_6 = F_6 C_6 + F_7 C_7$, since only a fraction, F_6, reaches stage 6 and an even smaller fraction, F_7, reaches stage 7. In general, the per capita cost at any given stage is the product of the unit cost, C_i, and the proportion of the target population that reach that stage, F_i. The cumulative per capita cost from stage i to the end is thus given by

$$A_i = \sum_{j=i}^{7} F_j C_j.$$

The total per capita cost of the entire program is then given by

$$K = A_1 = \sum_{j=1}^{7} F_j C_j.$$

The resource allocation, or cost-effectiveness, problem may be viewed in either of two ways. In one instance the decision maker might be faced with a constrained budget per capita, B. In that case, the object is to maximize effectiveness, E, subject to the constraint that per capita costs do not exceed the limit B. Formally, this problem is to

$$\text{maximize } E = p_1 p_2 p_3 p_4 p_5 p_6 p_7, \tag{6.1}$$

subject to the constraints

$$K = \sum_{i=1}^{7} F_i C_i \leqslant B, \tag{6.2}$$

and

$$0 \leqslant p_i \leqslant 1, \quad \text{for all } i. \tag{6.3}$$

An entirely equivalent formulation specifies a target level of effectiveness, E^*, and seeks to minimize the total costs of achieving that goal. In that case, the objective is to minimize

$$K = \sum_{i=1}^{7} F_i C_i, \tag{6.4}$$

subject to the constraints

$$E = p_1 p_2 p_3 p_4 p_5 p_6 p_7 \geqslant E^*, \tag{6.5}$$

and

$$0 \leqslant p_i \leqslant 1, \quad \text{for all } i. \tag{6.6}$$

In this analysis, the first formulation (expressions 6.1–6.3) is used. The analytical solution to this optimization problem is derived in the appendix to this chapter.

THE OPTIMAL CONDITIONS FOR RESOURCE ALLOCATION

Under the assumptions given regarding the shape of the cost functions, the optimality condition (that is, the equality that must hold if resources are being optimally allocated) is that the marginal cost of a proportional increase in effectiveness at any stage of the process must equal that of a proportional increase in effectiveness at any other stage of the process. As derived in the appendix to this chapter, the mathematical condition is that, for any two stages i and j,

$$F_{i+1}MC_i(p_i) + A_{i+1} = F_{j+1}MC_j(p_j) + A_{j+1},$$

where F_{i+1} is the cumulative probability of reaching stage $i+1$; $MC_i(p_i)$ is the marginal cost per unit increase in the probability (p_i) of progressing from stage i to stage $i+1$; and A_{i+1} is the total cost associated with all stages from the $(i+1)$th to the end of the process. Since $F_{i+1} = p_iF_i$, the above expression may be rewritten as

$$p_iF_iMC_i(p_i) + A_{i+1} = p_jF_jMC_j(p_j) + A_{j+1}. \qquad (6.7)$$

What can be learned from this equation to guide the allocation of resources to the detection and treatment of hypertension? The answer is quite a bit, even in the absence of hard data to give quantitative guidance to such allocation decisions. In particular, by interpreting each component of equation 6.7, one can derive strong reasons for favoring the allocation of resources to stages nearer the end of the process (for example, follow-up) rather than to stages nearer the beginning (for example, screening).

The focal points of equation 6.7 are the values of $MC_i(p_i)$ and $MC_j(p_j)$. These represent the marginal costs of achieving a unit increase in the transition probability from stage i to $i+1$ and from j to $j+1$ respectively. Thus, for example, if $MC_i(p_i) =$ \$1,000, then by definition the unit cost of achieving a percentage point improvement in the transition probability from stage i to stage $i+1$ is \$10 (or \$1,000/100). The higher $MC_i(p_i)$ is at the optimum, the greater the implied willingness to pay for an increment to the ith transition probability. If $MC_i(p_i)$ is larger than $MC_j(p_j)$ this means that the marginal percentage point change in the ith transition probability is costing more (that is, is worth more) than the marginal percentage point change in the ith transition probability. If the cost functions g_i and g_j were the same, then this would imply that the optimal situation (given the budget) is characterized by a higher level of p_i than of p_j.[4] For the reasons given below, it can indeed be expected that $MC_i(p_i)$ at the later stages will be larger than $MC_j(p_j)$ at the earlier stages and, hence, that relatively more effort should go into the later stages of the process.

---

4. Note that the function $MC_i(p_i)$ is the first derivative, or slope, of the cost function $g_i(p_i)$. Given the shape illustrated in figure 6.3, a higher slope implies a higher level of p_i.

Since the quantity $p_i F_i MC_i(p_i) + A_{i+1}$ from equation 6.7 is constant for all stages, the *lower* the values of F_i, A_{i+1}, or p_i, the *higher* will be the optimal level of $MC_i(p_i)$, and hence the *higher* will be the optimal level of p_i. This means that the greatest payoff for investment of resources lies in those stages for which (1) the cumulative probability of reaching the stage is relatively small, (2) the expected costs subsequent to the stage are relatively small, and (3) the base transition probability to the next stage is relatively small. All of these indications have sensible rationales, and all point to the desirability of channelling major resources to follow-up (S_6 and S_7) rather than to screening (S_2). They are considered one at a time in the following section.

INTERPRETATION OF THE OPTIMAL RESOURCE ALLOCATION CONDITIONS

In order to provide insight into the nature of optimal resource allocation in hypertension, the general solution to the optimization problem presented in the previous section must be interpreted. It was shown that, everything else being equal, more resources ought to go into improving adherence than into increasing initiation of treatment; more resources ought to go into increasing initiation of treatment than into ensuring referral to health care providers; and more resources ought to go into ensuring referral than into screening.

The first conclusion from the analysis was that the smaller the cumulative probability of reaching a given stage, the more valuable is an intervention to improve the performance of the system at that stage. This implies that interventions at the later stages, after most dropouts have already occurred, are more valuable than interventions at earlier stages. This stems from the fact that the unit cost of improving one of the probabilities in the chain must be multiplied by the number of people who have reached that stage. Since it makes no difference whether the improvement is in the first probability in the chain (screening) or in the last (adherence), the product of all the probabilities being the sole criterion, it is relatively cheaper to intervene after most of the attrition has already occurred.

The second conclusion was that the smaller the expected costs at stages subsequent to an intervention, the more valuable the intervention. This implies that interventions at later stages, after many of the costs have already been incurred, are more efficient than earlier interventions. If resources are spent increasing the rate of detection, costs will be incurred subsequently in referring, diagnosing, and treating many patients who will end up dropping out at various points along the way, never to be controlled. On the other hand, improvements in the rate of adherence will translate directly into benefits without any wasted costs subsequently. Those who make the final transition (that is, those who are controlled) have no further steps to take, and consequently the value of resources spent is fully realized.

The third conclusion was that the lower the base transition probability for a given stage, the more valuable is intervention to improve that probability. This implies that interventions at the weak links in the chain—those stages where the highest dropout rates occur—are the most valuable. Since the rate of adherence once treatment is initiated is generally believed to be one of the weakest links—less than 50 percent of patients adhere fully to medical regimens, compared to estimates of 50–60 percent who are aware of their hypertension and 50–70 percent who are treated once they are aware [Harris, 1973; Wilber and Barrow, 1972; Finnerty, Mattie, and Finnerty, 1973]—emphasis is logically placed on strengthening that link. Intuitively, since it is the *product* of the probabilities that determines effectiveness, equal proportional, not absolute, changes in the component probabilities yield equal benefit. Hence, the lower the initial level of the probability, the less the absolute increase required to yield equal benefit.

All of the above arguments favor allocating resources to improve retention and adherence (that is, increasing p_6 and p_7) over screening, even though, at first glance, screening may appear to be desirable because it is cheaper and is a "high yield" intervention. This makes it imperative that the effectiveness and costs of proadherence interventions be carefully evaluated. Even relatively modest benefits in these areas at relatively high costs may be better uses of limited resources than widespread screening and public education.

Calculation of Optimal Resource Allocation for a Hypothetical Hypertension Program

For illustrative purposes, the model developed and discussed above may be applied to the best available data from the literature to derive the optimal allocation of available resources in managing hypertension in a community. The data on transition probabilities, costs, and the cost functions relating the two represent best estimates.[5] Results support the conjecture made in the previous section by demonstrating the value of shifting resources from the front end of the system (screening) to the tail end (follow-up). Indeed, it is estimated that approximately a 40 percent increase in the number of hypertensives controlled could be achieved by such a reallocation.

The problem is defined as follows. A budget of $1,000,000 is available for a hypertension program. The objective is to allocate the budget among the first seven stages of the model represented in figure 6.1 in such a way as to maximize the number of hypertensives ultimately controlled.

Table 6.2 summarizes the baseline data on transition probabilities and costs for each of the stages. These data are baseline in the sense that possibilities for increasing probabilities by increasing expenditures at various stages are not yet included.

Entry into primary screening (S_1) is achieved at an education and outreach cost of $1 per capita. Primary screening (S_2) was assumed to cost $5 and to result in a 0.15 detection rate, based on a prevalence of 10 percent and a 33 percent false-positive rate. The cost figures were based on the $4 estimate by the American Heart Association [1974], adjusted upward to account for the fact that some door-to-door screens have been found to cost $10 or more [Taylor, 1975]. The prevalence rate approximates the fraction of United States adults with diastolic blood pressures above 95 mm Hg [National Center for Health Statistics, 1964a]. The fraction of false positives among all positives is a composite estimate from a variety of sources [Wilber and Barrow, 1972; Finnerty, Mattie, and Finnerty, 1973].

Referral of suspected hypertensives (S_3) was assumed to result in a 50 percent rate of appointments kept. This estimate was based on the study by Wilber and Barrow [1972], which found referral to vary from 45 percent to 59 percent depending on how the patient was notified about his high blood pressure. It was

---

5. Empirical studies would be useful in validating some of these data, to improve our confidence in the conclusions drawn from the model. Several such studies evaluating the cost-effectiveness of patient education interventions are being conducted under the auspices of the National High Blood Pressure Education Research Program, United States Department of Health, Education, and Welfare.

Table 6.2: Baseline costs and transition probabilities used in the analysis with the multistage model.

Stage number	Description	Unit cost (C_i)[a]	Transition probability (p_i)[b]
1	Target population	$ 1	
2	Screening	5	0.15
3	Suspected hypertension	0	.5
4	Secondary screening	15	.67
5	Confirmed hypertension	0	.75
6	Treatment begun	200	.67
7	Treatment continued	2800	.5
8	Controlled	—	—

[a] Cost per patient at stage i.
[b] Probability that a patient at stage i will reach stage $(i + 1)$.

assumed that referral requires no cost beyond that of screening, but cost functions introduced presently will allow for interventions to improve the referral rate at some cost.

The cost of secondary screening (S_4) was taken to be $15, reflecting additional pretreatment blood pressure readings. It was assumed that this procedure filters out the one-third of positives at primary screening who are not truly hypertensive.

Confirmation of the diagnosis (S_5) was assumed to result in initiation of therapy in 75 percent of all cases. This is based on the Harris study [1973] in which 76 percent of those who had been told they had hypertension said that their physicians had prescribed medication.

Initiation of treatment (S_6) was assumed to involve diagnostic evaluation followed by six months of therapy at a cost of $200 (see chapter 2 for the basis of this estimate), and to result in a dropout rate of one-third. The latter estimate was arrived at in two independent ways. First, the product of the last two transition rates $(p_5 \times p_6 = 3/4 \times 2/3 = 1/2)$ reflects the present situation in which one-half of known hypertensives are in continuing treatment [National High Blood Pressure Education Program, 1974]. Second, dropout rates of about one-third were found in programs in Atlanta (28 percent) [Wilber and Barrow, 1972] and Washington (42 percent) [Finnerty, Mattie, and Finnerty, 1973] in the absence of intensive follow-up interventions.

Continued lifetime treatment (S_7) was assumed to cost $2,800 (for an average 40-year-old, discounted at 5 percent per year, as derived in chapter 2), and to result in 50 percent of the patients having their blood pressures controlled (as stated by the National High Blood Pressure Education Program [1974] on the basis of several studies, for example, Wilber and Barrow [1972]). Both the dropout rate $(1 - p_6)$ and the adherence rate (p_7) are potentially subject to improvement if follow-up interventions are applied.

Budget allocations were computed first assuming that these baseline costs and probabilities apply, and then with costs and improvements in probabilities resulting from additional interventions. In the first case, in effect, the opportunity for "referral," "follow-up," and "continued follow-up" interventions to improve p_3, p_6, and p_7 respectively does not exist, or, if it does exist, it is bypassed in order to screen the maximum possible number of people. Under this maximum screening strategy, the total cost is computed as the baseline unit cost of each stage multiplied by the baseline proportion that reaches that stage, summed over all stages, and multiplied by the number screened. If x is the number screened, then the budget constraint is that

$$\$1,000,000 = x[\$1 + \$5 + (.15)(.5)\$15 + \\ (.15)(.5)(.67)(.75)\$200 + \\ (.15)(.5)(.67)(.75)(.67)\$2,800].$$

Thus, $x = 11,715$ are screened, but only 148 are controlled. This attrition process, together with the associated costs, is summarized in table 6.3, and serves as a point of comparison with the optimal allocation of resources.

Now consider the possibility that some of the transition prob-

Table 6.3: Budget allocation and attrition process for the "maximum screening" strategy.

Stage	Number entering	Cost
S_1 (target population)	11,715	$ 12,000
S_2 (screening)	11,715	59,000
S_3 (suspected hypertension)	1,757	0
S_4 (secondary screening)	879	13,000
S_5 (confirmed hypertension)	589	0
S_6 (treatment begun)	441	88,000
S_7 (treatment continued)	296	828,000
S_8 (controlled)	148	$1,000,000 (total)

abilities can be improved by increasing the unit costs at certain stages. Emphasis is placed on the probability of referral to secondary screening (p_3), of not dropping out of treatment once it is begun (p_6), and of adherence and control (p_7). Interventions at these stages may include intensive referral efforts, improved access to care, and patient education, respectively. The possibility of improving the probability that a newly confirmed hypertensive enters treatment (p_5)—for example, through professional education—might also have been considered but was not. Interventions that would affect two or more transition probabilities simultaneously were also excluded. Table 6.4 describes the assumed incremental costs of three hypothetical interventions and the resulting improvements in the corresponding transition rates.

In the case of referral of suspected hypertensives (C_3, p_3), it was assumed that an additional expenditure of $50 per capita (for example, through efforts of screeners to schedule appointments for patients with providers or to ensure that appointments are made by the patients themselves) would cut the nonreferral

Table 6.4: Costs and yields of referral and follow-up interventions.

(1) Transition probability	(2) Intervention	(3) Base unit cost ($)[a]	(4) Increment in unit cost ($) to reduce attrition by half[b]	(5) Base probability[c]	(6) Achieved probability[d]
p_3	Increase referral of suspected hypertensives	0	50	0.50	0.75
p_6	Facilitate continuation of treatment once begun	200	100	.67	.83
p_7	Improve adherence to continued treatment	2800	350	.50	.75

[a] Cost per patient at this stage in the absence of additional intervention (see table 6.2).

[b] Incremental cost per patient at this stage required to reduce attrition between this stage and the next by half.

[c] Probability that a patient at this stage will reach the next stage in the absence of additional intervention.

[d] Probability that a patient at this stage will reach the next stage with the intervention at the cost given in column (4). Equals (1 + base probability) ÷ 2.

rate in half, thus increasing the referral rate from 0.50 to 0.75. This assumption is supported by the experience of Finnerty, Mattie, and Finnerty [1973].

In the case of continuation of treatment once begun (C_6, p_6), it was assumed that an additional expenditure of $100 during the first year (for example, for more frequent office visits, patient education, or improved access or convenience) would cut the dropout rate in half, thus increasing the retention rate from 0.67 to 0.83. This too is supported by the experience of Finnerty's program, which reduced the dropout rate to 17 percent by providing, among other things, an increased frequency of office visits in the first six months of treatment.

Finally, for continued treatment (C_7, p_7), it was assumed that an additional expenditure of $25 per year, or a present value of $350 over the lifetime of therapy (for example, for counseling or patient education) would cut the nonadherence rate in half, thus increasing the rate of control from 0.50 to 0.75. This assumption is largely speculative, but reflects the anticipated improvements being built into several studies of the effectiveness of patient education, and a cost equivalent to about two extra physician visits per year.

Cost functions of the shape illustrated in figure 6.5 were estimated for each of these three stages. This was done by fitting the baseline and achieved combinations of unit cost and probability from table 6.4 to curves of the form

$$g_i(p_i) = a_i + b_i/(1 - p_i), \qquad \text{for } p_i \geqslant p_i^*,$$

where a_i and b_i are the parameters to be calculated, p_i^* is the "base" transition probability in the absence of any follow-up intervention, and p_i is the probability achieved. This functional form was chosen arbitrarily to reflect increasing marginal costs of improving the probabilities, and to become unbounded as the probability nears the ideal value of unity. The fitted cost functions are shown in figure 6.6 along with the fixed cost functions for the other transition probabilities.

The optimal budget allocation given these cost functions was derived from the optimality conditions in equation 6.7. The variables subject to choice are C_3, the unit cost devoted to improving referral; C_6, the unit cost devoted to initiating treatment and preliminary efforts to achieve continued care; C_7, the unit cost devoted to continued proadherence interventions; and x,

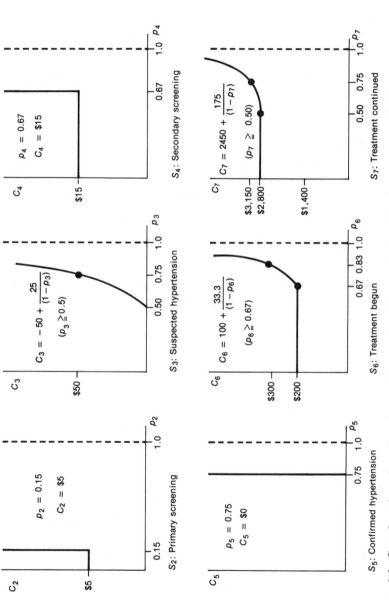

Figure 6.6: Cost functions for selected transition probabilities, including the effects of interventions to alter them.

the number of people brought into screening. The remaining costs and probabilities are not subject to choice.

Based upon these conditions the optimal allocation of the budget of $1,000,000 has the following characteristics: the adherence rate is increased to 0.81 by adding $571 to the unit cost of lifetime treatment for continued follow-up; the initial dropout rate is reduced to 0.24 by adding $39 to the unit cost of therapy in the first year for patient-oriented activities; the referral rate is held at 0.50, resources not being profitably applied at that stage;[6] 8,875 people are screened, compared to 11,715 under the maximum screening strategy, a decrease of 24 percent; 206 hypertensives are controlled, compared to only 148 under the maximum screening strategy, an improvement of 39 percent. The division of the budget and the attrition process under the optimal strategy are shown in table 6.5.

There are two major observations to be made on the basis of these results. The first is that they confirm numerically the proposition derived theoretically in the previous section that the amount we should be willing to pay per person to improve the transition probabilities at the end stages of the process (that is, adherence) is substantially greater than the amount we should be willing to pay per person to improve the transition probabilities at

Table 6.5: Budget allocation and attrition process for the "optimal" strategy.[a]

Stage	Number entering	Cost (nearest thousand)
S_1 (target population)	8,875	$ 9,000
S_2 (screening)	8,875	44,000
S_3 (suspected hypertension)	1,331	0
S_4 (secondary screening)	666	10,000
S_5 (confirmed hypertension)	446	0
S_6 (treatment begun)	335	80,000[b]
S_7 (treatment continued)	254	857,000[c]
S_8 (controlled)	206	$1,000,000 (total)

[a] Based on the costs and yields of interventions specified in table 6.4.
[b] Includes $39 additional per capita for follow-up.
[c] Includes $571 additional per capita for enhanced follow-up.

6. This is a corner solution, the optimality conditions (equation 6.7) having yielded a value of $p_3 < 0.5$.

the front end (that is, detection). One measure of this is the marginal cost of achieving the last percentage point improvement in the probabilities at each stage, a higher marginal cost at the optimum indicating a greater willingness to pay for the change in probability. At stage 1, this marginal cost is $0.01; at stage 3 it is $1.00; at stage 6 it is $6.29; and at stage 7 it is $48.48. Thus, even though a dollar per patient at stage 3 yields nearly 50 times as great an increase in the respective transition probability as at stage 7, that dollar per patient is still better spent at stage 7, and while it is extremely cheap to get people through the early stages, it is still a better use of resources to screen fewer people and apply what appears to be an expensive follow-up program to those who reach treatment.

The second observation is that the optimal strategy significantly increases the number of patients controlled per unit expenditure compared to the maximum screening strategy. Alternatively stated, the cost per patient controlled is about $5,000 under the optimal strategy, compared to $7,000 under the maximum screening strategy. This suggests that even if we do not choose to allocate *more* resources to hypertension control, it is plausible that significant improvements in efficiency can be achieved by shifting existing resources.

The data on which these findings are based undoubtedly do not apply to all health care settings. In some, serious institutional or political considerations may make screening a relatively more favored activity than efficiency criteria would suggest. Nonetheless, the magnitude of the potential health benefits to be derived mandate efforts to change from the current propensity toward widespread screening to more intensive efforts to improve adherence.

Sensitivity Analysis

Recognizing that the cost functions describing potential improvements in referral, retention, and adherence are somewhat speculative and are based on limited evidence, it is important to determine how sensitive the findings are to those assumptions. To that end, a sensitivity analysis was performed that varied the parameters of the cost functions in the direction unfavorable to follow-up until the optimum shifted in favor of the maximum screening strategy.

First the three interventions intended to improve referral (p_3), retention (p_6), and adherence (p_7), respectively, were assumed to be substantially less effective than the parameters in table 6.4 indicate. For each, the specified incremental costs were assumed to purchase only a 20 percent reduction in attrition instead of 50 percent. Thus, $350 in additional continued follow-up costs (C_7) was assumed to improve adherence (p_7) from 0.50 to 0.60, rather than to 0.75. This is equivalent to an increase in follow-up costs from $350 to $1,200 for achieving the original 50 percent improvement (figure 6.6).

The nature of the optimal strategy, emphasizing long-term follow-up, was robust under these changed assumptions. While it was no longer cost-effective to apply additional resources to efforts to avoid dropouts (p_6), an additional expenditure of $659 per patient on continued follow-up and proadherence measures was indicated, raising the adherence rate from 0.50 to 0.66. The complete budget allocation is shown in table 6.6. A total of 163 patients could be controlled under the budget, compared to 148 under the maximum screening strategy. While this improvement is not as dramatic as that found in the original analysis, it is significant that a substantially less favorable set of assumptions concerning the cost-effectiveness of follow-up failed to turn the tide to the maximum screening strategy. The number screened under these assumptions is, however, greater than under the original assumptions, reflecting the higher residual dropout and

Table 6.6: Budget allocation and attrition process for the optimal strategy: sensitivity analysis.[a]

Stage	Number entering	Cost (nearest thousand)
S_1 (target population)	9,803	$ 10,000
S_2 (screening)	9,803	49,000
S_3 (suspected hypertension)	1,471	0
S_4 (secondary screening)	735	11,000
S_5 (confirmed hypertension)	493	0
S_6 (treatment begun)	369	74,000
S_7 (treatment continued)	248	856,000[b]
S_8 (controlled)	163	$1,000,000 (total)

[a] Assuming that a proadherence intervention costing $350 per patient reduces nonadherence by 20 percent, rather than 50 percent.
[b] Includes $659 additional per capita for enhanced follow-up.

nonadherence rates despite the increased per capita expenditure on follow-up.

In a second sensitivity analysis, the cost-effectiveness of enhanced follow-up was assumed to be even worse. A per capita expenditure of $350 was assumed to purchase a reduction in nonadherence of only 10 percent. In effect, the follow-up intervention was assumed to be a very expensive vehicle for achieving a very small reduction in attrition. Under these conditions, the intervention did cease to be cost-effective, and maximum screening became optimal. This result required a very striking decrease in the effectiveness of the interventions, however.

A third sensitivity analysis assumed that primary screening is essentially costless ($C_2 = 0$), but that the other costs and probabilities are as originally specified. Despite this assumption favorable to screening, the optimal strategy remained the same, calling for $571 in additional per-patient expenditures to increase the adherence rate to 0.81. Under the optimal strategy, 9,332 persons would be screened and 215 thereby controlled. This is still far superior to the maximum screening strategy, which results in 12,599 screened but only 157 controlled.

A final sensitivity analysis, examining the effects of increasing the assumed prevalence of hypertension in the target population from 10 percent to 20 percent and thus increasing the value of p_2 from 0.15 to 0.30, was also performed. All other parameters were kept at their original values (tables 6.2 and 6.4). Under the maximum screening strategy, 6,094 individuals were screened and 153 ultimately were controlled. The optimal strategy called for a per-patient proadherence expenditure of $571 (as was the case with the 10 percent prevalence rate), thus increasing adherence (p_7) from 0.50 to 0.81. The dropout rate ($1 - p_6$) was reduced to 0.27 by an additional per-patient expenditure of $23. A total of 4,684 individuals were screened, and 212 were controlled, again for an improvement of almost 40 percent over the maximum screening strategy. Thus, even in populations with a relatively high prevalence of hypertension (for example, black communities), where screening might be expected to be most cost-effective, these results suggest that interventions to reduce the number of dropouts and to improve adherence should be emphasized.

In the spirit of sensitivity analysis, the necessary and sufficient conditions under which each strategy would dominate were com-

puted. This allows the cost functions for improving the performance of the system at various stages to be left unspecified
and allows the characteristics of those functions that would
support the status quo allocation of resources to follow-up to be
assessed. Using the baseline probabilities in table 6.2, for the
maximum screening strategy to be optimal (that is, screening,
diagnosis, and treatment with no additional follow-up), the per-
patient marginal cost of increasing the adherence probability by
one percentage point must be at least $67.70. This is derived as
80 percent of the average cost of primary screening, *plus* 6 percent of the average cost of secondary screening, *plus* 3 percent of
the average first-year cost of diagnosis and treatment, *plus* 2 percent of the average lifetime cost of continued treatment, *plus*
$0.80.[7] Any smaller per-patient cost of increasing adherence by
one percentage point implies that at least some additional resources are wisely spent on improving adherence.

Research and Development in Follow-up
and Proadherence Interventions

It has been shown that if interventions are available that even
remotely approach the cost-effectiveness of those described in
table 6.4, then more follow-up and less screening is the optimal
course of action. If, however, such interventions are not widely
available, or if the cost-effectiveness of those currently available
is as poor as hypothesized in the second sensitivity analysis, the
policy question arises whether it is worth investing in research
efforts to develop and generalize methods to improve adherence.
The federal government, through the National High Blood Pressure Education Research Program, has undertaken research along
these lines. The question remains, however, if major national
resources are to be devoted to hypertension programs, is the

---

7. From equation 6.7,
$$p_1 MC_1(p_1) + A_2 = p_7 F_7 MC_7(p_7) + A_8.$$
Simplification and substitution lead to
$$MC_7(p_7) = (1/F_8)[MC_1(p_1) + F_2 C_2 + F_3 C_3 + F_4 C_4 + F_5 C_5 + F_6 C_6 + F_7 C_7].$$
Since the marginal cost of a one percentage point increase in adherence is
$MC_7(p_7)/100$, and baseline $F_8 = 0.0125$, and the other F_i are as derived from
table 6.2, the necessary and sufficient condition for the baseline to be optimal
is that the marginal cost of a one percentage point increase exceed
$$.8[MC_1(p_1) + C_2 + .15C_3 + .075C_4 + .05C_5 + .0375C_6 + .025C_7].$$
Since by assumption $C_3 = C_5 = 0$, the result in the text is obtained.

amount we are spending on research to improve adherence enough?

A sense of the answer to this question can be had by considering how much of the million dollar budget in the analysis we would be willing to devote to developing that intervention. If the status quo yields 148 controlled hypertensives for every million dollars (table 6.3), and the new technology yields 206 controlled hypertensives, then we can devote *one-quarter* of the total budget to research and still be ahead, provided that research led to the development of effective interventions. This is so because three-quarters of a million dollars results in the control of 75% $\times$ 206 = 154 hypertensives, more than the 148 controlled for the full million dollars under the status quo. This exercise in fact *understates* the value of the research since the intervention, once developed, is available in perpetuity to yield dividends for future cohorts of new hypertensives as well as for those currently in the target population.

Optimal policy is likely to involve a greater proportional commitment to such research than is now being pursued. It may even be best to postpone some screening and treatment efforts until interventions exist that would make such programs significantly more cost-effective. The tradeoff between realizing benefits from the expenditure of health dollars on cost-effective programs today, and waiting until those dollars can yield even more benefits per dollar spent in the future, is a classic case of foregoing immediate consumption of benefit in order to invest in even more future consumption. Even if technologies did exist that approximated the cost-effectiveness of those hypothesized in the analysis, it still might be worth making the investment to improve their cost-effectiveness further. A premium of $350 to increase one's likelihood of adhering to a course of therapy from 50 percent to 75 percent or even to 60 percent might be worth paying, but further research might lead to even more effective and less costly interventions. If, for example, methods of public education, including school health programs, could be developed to effectively change attitudes toward health care, then adherence might improve to the point that it would cease to be the major problem it is today. Clearly, while present knowledge suggests a reallocation of resources from screening to follow-up, a major fraction of resources allocated to hypertension should be devoted to programs of research and development of innovative and cost-effective approaches to improving adherence.

Appendix to Chapter 6

The general resource allocation problem is to maximize

$$E = F_{n+1} = \prod_{i=1}^{n} p_i \tag{6A.1}$$

subject to the constraints

$$K = \sum_{i=1}^{n} F_i C_i \leqslant B \tag{6A.2}$$

and

$$0 \leqslant p_i \leqslant 1, \quad \text{for all } i, \tag{6A.3}$$

as developed in the text. For the model shown in figure 6.1, $n = 7$.

It is assumed for now that the cost functions $C_i = g_i(p_i)$ are strictly increasing everywhere, $g_i'(p_i) > 0$, and that they exhibit increasing marginal cost, $g_i''(p_i) > 0$, in the relevant range. The cost function illustrated in figure 6.3 is of this type. These assumptions will be relaxed presently.

The optimality conditions are derived by adjoining the constraint (6A.2) to the maximand (6A.1), differentiating with respect to each p_i, and setting the results to zero. The Lagrangean is given by

$$L = \prod_{i=1}^{n} p_i - \lambda \left[\sum_{i=1}^{n} (\prod_{j=0}^{i-1} p_j) g_i(p_i) - B \right].$$

Proceeding inductively,

$$\frac{\partial L}{\partial p_n} = F_n - \lambda F_n g_n'(p_n) = 0 ,$$

so that

$$\lambda = 1/g_n'(p_n) . \tag{6A.4}$$

Thus, the shadow price, λ, of the budget constraint (that is, the value of an extra dollar in improving program effectiveness) is equal to the increment achievable in the final transition probability in the chain. Continuing inductively,

$$\frac{\partial L}{\partial p_{n-1}} = F_{n+1}/p_{n-1} - \lambda F_{n-1}g'_{n-1}(p_{n-1}) - \lambda F_n g_n(p_n)/p_{n-1} = 0.$$

Multiplying through by p_{n-1}, and substituting from equation 6A.4, the following result obtains:

$$F_{n+1}g'_n(p_n) = F_n g'_{n-1}(p_{n-1}) + F_n g_n(p_n). \qquad (6A.5)$$

Recognizing that $F_n g_n(p_n) = F_n C_n = A_n$ is the cost from stage n to the end of the process (the end being stage $n + 1$), and recognizing that $A_{n+1} = 0$, we may foresee the general result (equation 6.7 in the text) and write 6A.5 as

$$F_{n+1}g'_n(p_n) + A_{n+1} = F_n g'_{n-1}(p_{n-1}) + A_n . \qquad (6A.6)$$

It is straightforward to demonstrate inductively that equation 6A.6 holds more generally; that is,

$$F_{i+1}g'_i(p_i) + A_{i+1} = F_{j+1}g'_j(p_j) + A_{j+1} , \qquad \text{all } i, j = 1, \ldots, n. \qquad (6A.7)$$

The interpretation of this result gives insight into the rationale for optimal resource allocation, and is discussed in the text.[1]

Next, consider the implications of relaxing some of the stringent assumptions in order to make the model more realistic and generally applicable. In particular, the assumption that the cost functions are of the type shown in figure 6.3 may not be appropriate. A possibly more realistic assumption for many of the transition probabilities is as illustrated by figure 6.5. This formulation posits a base transition probability p_i^*, associated with a base cost C_i^*, with improvements in p_i being achievable at an increase in cost above the base level. It is still assumed that the convexity conditions, $g''_i(p_i) > 0$, hold for $p_i > p_i^*$.

The implication of these revised assumptions is to introduce the possibility of a corner solution, that is, an allocation in which the optimal thing to do is to achieve the "minimum" transition rate p_i^* for one or more stages. For such stages, the optimality condition (6A.7) would not hold, and would be replaced by an analogous equation involving the shadow price of the "quasi-

---

1. Since $g'_i(p_i)$ is the marginal cost $MC_i(p_i)$ as defined in the text, equation 6A.7 is identical to equation 6.7 in the text as claimed.

constraint" $p_i \geqslant p_i^*$. However, the essential character of the optimal solution in the fully convex case, that is, where $g_i''(p_i)$ are everywhere positive, carries over to the more realistic case as well, and consequently the interpretive discussion in the text remains valid. The numerical example developed in the text using cost functions of this form does involve corner solutions.

7. Evaluation of Specific Causes of Hypertension: Cost-Effectiveness Considerations

Though a great deal has been learned about the epidemiology and pathophysiology of hypertension, the fundamental cause in the vast majority of patients remains unknown. As a result, therapy is directed at the major external manifestation of the condition, elevated blood pressure. In a minority of patients, however, ranging from an estimated 1 percent in a population sample [Taylor, 1974] to greater than 10 percent in referral practices [Gifford, 1969], definitive causal mechanisms—"secondary causes"—can be defined. Specific, curative therapy can be applied in perhaps half of such cases.

To determine the extent to which diagnostic evaluation for specific causes of hypertension is indicated on the basis of cost-effectiveness, both the effectiveness and risks of diagnostic procedures and the benefits and risks of alternative modes of therapy must be evaluated in relation to their costs. Because the ultimate objective of treatment is, of course, to maximize both survival and quality of life of patients afflicted with hypertension, physicians often argue that the best medical treatment should be provided regardless of cost. From the point of view of society, however, the incremental cost and benefit provided by one mode of therapy over another must also be considered.

Causes of Secondary Hypertension

The causes of secondary hypertension separate into those for which specific modes of therapy are currently available and those for which treatment is primarily nonspecific and consists of anti-

---

Note: The authors of this chapter are Barbara J. McNeil, William B. Stason, and Milton C. Weinstein.

hypertensive medications. Even for the latter, however, despite the absence of specific modes of therapy, knowledge of causation may be important in predicting prognosis and anticipating potential complications and drug side effects.

Adequate data on the prevalence of secondary causes of hypertension are not available in the literature. Those that do exist are derived from academic centers to which patients with difficult or enigmatic hypertension problems are referred. These statistics, therefore, measure prevalence in highly selected populations and, in all probability, overestimate the true prevalence of certain causes of secondary hypertension by a considerable factor. Among the best data are those from the Cleveland Clinics, where a total of 4,939 patients with hypertension were examined during 1966–1967 [Gifford, 1969]. The diagnostic breakdown of these was as follows:

> *Specific therapy available*
> Renovascular disease: 220 (4.5%); operated: 67 (1.4%)
> Coarctation of the aorta: 30 (0.6%)
> Primary hyperaldosteronism: 20 (0.4%)
> Pheochromocytoma: 9 (0.2%)
> Cushing's disease: 11 (0.2%)
>
> *No specific therapy available*
> Primary hypertension: 4,392 (89%)
> Chronic glomerulonephritis (chronic renal disease): 257 (5.2%)

Hence, specific therapeutic interventions were potentially available for only 5.9 percent of hypertensive patients and apparently applied in 2.8 percent or less. If this were a population-based sample rather than one from a referral center, these prevalences would undoubtedly be considerably lower.

A cause of reversible hypertension, which is not included in the above list but has attracted considerable attention in recent years, is associated with the ingestion of oral contraceptives. Seven to fifteen percent of women taking oral contraceptives develop high blood pressure [Ayers et al., 1973]. In the vast majority, blood pressure returns to normal within four to six months after discontinuing the medication. For these patients, diagnosis and treatment consist only of a careful history and a period of observation off contraceptives.

Screening for Secondary Hypertension

The diagnostic evaluation of a patient with established hypertension includes a medical history aimed at delineating symptoms that suggest either a specific cause or adverse effects of the hypertension; a physical examination to identify salient physical manifestations; and laboratory examinations. The latter have three primary objectives: to facilitate clinical management by ascertaining the degree of damage to the cardiovascular system, kidneys, or eyes; to serve as baselines for monitoring side effects from antihypertensive medications; and to screen for possible secondary causes of hypertension. Confirmatory diagnostic tests or procedures are then performed on patients whose screening test results are abnormal.

This chapter focuses on the cost and effectiveness considerations involved in screening for secondary hypertension and presents a detailed analysis for the most important of these conditions, renovascular disease.

CRITERIA FOR SCREENING

The efficiency of screening for secondary hypertension depends on several factors. The most important of these are: (1) the availability of a sensitive, specific, and inexpensive screening test; (2) a relatively high prevalence of the condition in question; and (3) the availability of a specific therapeutic intervention that can result in better health outcomes or lower cost than alternative modes of therapy. These factors are different for each cause of secondary hypertension.

CHRONIC RENAL DISEASE

Hypertension may be the result of kidney failure stemming from a number of acquired and congenital abnormalities. Chronic pyelonephritis, resulting from recurrent kidney infections, and glomerulonephritis, an immune disease frequently occurring as an aftermath of streptococcal infections, are the most common. Predisposing congenital conditions include polycystic kidneys, hereditary nephritis, and glomerulosclerosis (a form of kidney disease that occurs with increased frequency in diabetics). Specific therapy for these conditions, either to forestall progression of the renal damage or to relieve associated hypertension, is rarely available, but the diagnosis is useful to identify the need for renal dialysis or kidney transplantation when the renal failure is far advanced, and to provide a prognosis.

COARCTATION OF THE AORTA

Coarctation of the aorta is a congenital narrowing of the major blood vessel leading from the heart (aorta). It is a frequent cause of hypertension in children but rarely goes undetected into adult life. Because it is readily detected in a routine physical examination, it presents little problem in diagnosis. Surgical treatment to relieve the narrowing of the aorta is the preferred treatment and has been clearly shown to improve the natural history of the condition [Schuster and Gross, 1962]. Whether antihypertensive medications would be equally effective is not known because no clinical trials involving their use have been performed. It is unlikely, however, that such treatment would relieve the symptoms of insufficient blood supply to the legs that frequently accompany coarctation of the aorta.

CUSHING'S DISEASE

Cushing's disease is an endocrine disorder resulting from overproduction of certain hormones by a tumor or by excessive activity (hyperplasia) of the adrenal glands. Hypertension is but one manifestation of a symptom complex that includes obesity, osteopososis (thin bones), diabetes mellitus, facial plethora (redness), hirsutism (excessive body hair), and sexual malfunction. These symptoms usually lead to ready identification of the condition. Laboratory examinations are used to verify its presence. Because of its distinctive features and its rarity, Cushing's disease does not present a major problem in screening a hypertensive population. Surgical removal of the tumor or adrenal glands is successful in controlling the disease and its associated hypertension in most patients.

PRIMARY ALDOSTERONISM

Primary aldosteronism results from overproduction of the salt-retaining hormone, aldosterone, by either a benign tumor (adenoma) or excessive activity (bilateral hyperplasia) of the adrenal glands. This disease has stirred a great deal of interest among medical researchers because of the important contributions its study has made to our understanding of the pathophysiology of hypertension.

Symptoms, if present, are relatively nonspecific and include weakness and excessive urination. Blood pressure elevations are only moderate, and severe hypertension is extremely rare. The diagnosis is usually suspected when a low serum potassium level (hypokalemia) is found incidentally at the time of initial evaluation. Because this test has a very high incidence of both false-positive and false-negative results, several alternative diagnostic strategies can be considered once hypokalemia is found. These include:

• Repeat the serum potassium with the patient off antihypertensive medications and proceed with confirmatory tests only if hypokalemia is verified.

• Proceed directly with urinary potassium determinations and measurements of plasma renin activity and plasma aldosterone. Such tests, if positive, usually lead to hospitalization for extensive metabolic balance studies. If the preliminary examinations are performed carefully in a stepwise fashion, however, the need for hospitalization can be limited to the very small group of patients in whom the diagnosis is most likely.

• Begin antihypertensive therapy directly, avoiding drugs that tend to lower serum potassium further and monitoring serum potassium closely. Proceed with further diagnostic studies and specific surgical treatment only if medical therapy is unsuccessful. The risk of delaying specific therapy is minimal provided these precautions are taken.

Because of the low prevalence of primary aldosteronism, its relatively benign character, the complex nature of laboratory examinations necessary to verify its presence, and the availability of effective alternative treatment for at least a proportion of patients, vigorous pursuit of its diagnosis in a general hypertensive population is unlikely to be cost-effective.

PHEOCHROMOCYTOMA

This rare tumor of the adrenal gland or sympathetic nervous system secretes excessive catecholamines (hormones that tend to increase blood pressure) and causes a form of hypertension with unique characteristics [Levine and Landsberg, 1974; Kaplan, 1973]. Like primary aldosteronism, it is very rare, occurring at

202 Hypertension: A Policy Perspective

the very most in 0.5 percent of the adult hypertensive population. Unlike primary aldosteronism, however, it is frequently associated with troublesome symptoms (headaches, nervousness, sweating, and palpitations) and severe hypertension. Hypertensive paroxysms or crises occur and may lead to malignant hypertension, cerebral hemorrhage, or cardiac arrhythmia, each carrying a significant risk of death. Treatment with the usual antihypertensive agents is seldom successful in controlling the blood pressure and may even result in paradoxical increases. Specific medical and surgical treatments can cure or control the disease in a majority of patients at reasonable risks. For these reasons, the "cost of delay" in establishing the diagnosis may be considerable.

Against these considerations must be balanced the costs of screening for an extremely rare disease. If proper precautions are applied, available screening tests are both sensitive (true-positive ratio greater than 90 percent) and specific (false-positive ratio less than 10 percent). With a condition as rare as this, however, the false-positive rate must be extremely low to avoid a large number of unnecessary evaluations of misdiagnosed patients.

Strategies that have been proposed include:

• Screen all hypertensives despite the disease's low prevalence.
• Screen only those hypertensives who present with symptoms suggestive of pheochromocytoma. This strategy limits screening to about 10 percent of the hypertensive population while running the risk of missing the approximately 10 percent of patients with pheochromocytoma who have no symptoms.
• Screen only those hypertensives whose symptoms and blood pressures are not controlled by antihypertensive medications. This strategy, while perhaps a more efficient use of diagnostic resources, suffers from the risks associated with delaying or missing the diagnosis.

Each of these strategies has different implications in terms of cost-effectiveness. The basic tradeoff is between the marginal cost of establishing the diagnosis and the risk of delaying the diagnosis and implementation of specific therapy. Most experts recommend erring on the side of "medical conservatism." Of all the causes of secondary hypertension for which screening and specific therapy are available, pheochromocytoma is the one for which the greatest consensus exists that screening should be done [Ayers et al., 1973]. Nevertheless, a cost-effectiveness analysis based on realistic population-based prevalence data may indicate that even for this dangerous condition, selective screening based on symptoms or nonresponse to antihypertensive therapy is preferred to widespread screening.

RENOVASCULAR DISEASE

Renovascular disease (RVD) is the most frequent cause of secondary hypertension for which specific corrective treatment is available. Prevalence estimates in the selected populations of referral centers range from 4.5 percent [Gifford, 1969] to as high as 10 percent [Laragh, 1972]. RVD causes narrowing of one or both renal arteries, which leads to a diminished blood supply to the kidney(s) and to systemic hypertension. Alterations in relationships among the hormones renin, angiotensin, and aldosterone appear to be responsible for the elevations in blood pressure. Etiologically, RVD can be divided broadly into fibromuscular hyperplasia (FM), which affects women 4 or 5 times as frequently as men and has a mean age of diagnosis in the fifth decade, and arteriosclerosis (AS), which affects men slightly more frequently (3 to 2) and is most common in the sixth decade [Maxwell et al., 1972]. Only rarely are there specific symptoms or physical manifestations to suggest the diagnosis.

Surgical interventions to correct or bypass the obstruction in the renal artery (or arteries) or to remove the ischemic (blood-deficient) kidney can be offered to many patients. The Cooperative Study on Renovascular Disease indicated that cure, defined as reduction of diastolic blood pressure to 90 mm Hg or less and 10 mm Hg less than the preoperative level one year postoperatively, occurred in 58 percent of patients with FM and 40 percent of those with AS [Foster, Maxwell, and Franklin, 1975]. Operative mortality was 3.4 percent in the former group and 9.3 percent in the latter [Franklin et al., 1975].

Despite the availability of radiologic screening examinations and surgical procedures to achieve cure, optimal management of this condition remains problematic because of the good blood pressure control achieved in many patients with antihypertensive medications. Under these conditions a careful assessment of benefits, risks, and costs of alternative strategies is particularly critical.

SCREENING FOR RENOVASCULAR DISEASE.   Confronted with a hypertensive population, the initial question is whether to screen for RVD and, if so, whether to screen the entire population or a subgroup selected on the basis of age, sex, and clinical findings. The most frequently employed screening test is hypertensive intravenous pyelography (IVP), an x-ray procedure that assesses both the structure and function of the kidneys. For patients with an abnormal IVP, renal arteriography and renal vein renin measurements are required to confirm the presence of RVD and to indicate whether it is of the fibromuscular or arteriosclerotic type. The decision to proceed with surgical treatment depends on the results.

Two diagnostic strategies are presented diagrammatically in figure 7.1 [McNeil and Adelstein, 1975]. In strategy 1, all patients are screened for RVD with an IVP and, if this is abnormal, further examinations are performed. Surgery is then given to all patients with confirmed FM and to those with AS who are considered to be operable. The balance with AS are treated medically. In strategy 2, no one is screened, and medical treatment is given to all patients. An intermediate strategy would be that of targeted screening for those at highest risk of RVD.

Outcomes associated with medical or surgical management are depicted in figure 7.2. A patient who undergoes surgery has a finite risk of operative mortality. Survivors may be "cured" or "not cured." If the latter, they are given medical treatment with the effectiveness depicted at C_1 and C_2. These responses are influenced by a patient's pharmacologic responsiveness to medications, by the adequacy of doses prescribed, and by adherence to the prescribed regimen. The terminal branches of this decision diagram show the possible outcomes: the patient may remain well without complications, suffer impairments of health status due to nonfatal morbid events (chiefly strokes and heart attacks) or side effects of medications, or he may die.

COST-EFFECTIVENESS ANALYSIS.   This analysis considers the cost-effectiveness of diagnostic testing of the entire hypertensive population in a given age-sex cohort (strategy 1), relative to that for universal medical antihypertensive management (strategy 2). The advantages of strategy 1 (IVP/surgery)—its ability to achieve blood pressure reduction without the side effects of medications or the problems of adherence associated with medical therapy—are balanced against the risk of surgical mortality and the high cost of specific diagnosis and surgical cure. Because the optimal choice depends on the age and sex of the patient (for example, a preference for surgery in younger patients), the

STRATEGY 1

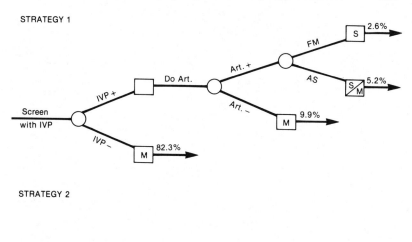

STRATEGY 2

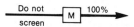

Figure 7.1: Decision flow diagrams for the diagnosis and treatment of patients with hypertension. Squares denote decision nodes, and circles chance nodes. The alternate paths for each decision node are not shown; rather, the decision nodes indicate the one selected. **Strategy 1:** Screening is performed on all patients with hypertension. If the intravenous pyelogram (IVP) is abnormal (IVP+), arteriography (Art) is always performed. When the IVP or arteriogram is negative, medical therapy (M) is followed. When the arteriogram is positive (Art+) and patients are found to have fibromuscular (FM) disease, surgical treatment is chosen (S). When they are found to have arteriosclerotic (AS) disease, surgical or medical treatment (S/M) may be chosen. **Strategy 2:** No screening with intravenous pyelography is done, and all patients are treated medically (M). (Source: McNeil and Adelstein [1975].)

analysis is carried out for men and women aged 30 and 50. Two surgical substrategies are considered. In the first, surgery is given only to patients with fibromuscular disease; in the second, surgery is given to those with either fibromuscular hyperplasia (FM) or arteriosclerotic disease (AS). The former leads to a lower surgical mortality rate but has the disadvantage of a higher cost of finding a candidate for surgery. The pretreatment diastolic blood pressure is assumed to be 110 mm Hg, controllable to 90 mm Hg with therapy.

Data base. Hypertensive subjects to whom the analysis refers are those 24 million Americans with diastolic blood pressures greater than 160/95 mm Hg. Data from the Cooperative Study of Renovascular Disease for patients with either RVD or essential

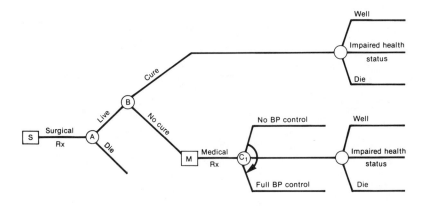

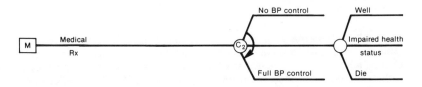

Figure 7.2: Outcomes associated with the surgical and medical regimens.
The results of surgical management of patients with renovascular disease
are detailed at chance nodes A and B. Results of primary or supplemental
medical therapy are expressed at nodes C_1 and C_2. All other terminal
chance nodes are associated with possible outcomes ranging from good
health, to varying degrees of impaired health status, to death.

hypertension serve as the basis for calculations [Maxwell et al.,
1972; Foster, Maxwell, and Franklin, 1975; Franklin et al.,
1975]. As an upper bound, the prevalence of RVD was taken to
be 10 percent [Laragh, 1972]. The age- and sex-specific proportions of FM and AS among those with RVD were based on the
Cooperative Study [Maxwell et al., 1972]. As shown in table 7.1,
these proportions vary considerably.

Surgical cure rates and operative mortality rates were taken
from the Cooperative Study [Foster, Maxwell, and Franklin,
1975; Franklin et al., 1975]. Under the criterion for abnormality
chosen by that study [Bookstein et al., 1972], 78 percent of
patients with RVD had an abnormal IVP (true-positive ratio,
0.78) and 11 percent who ultimately proved not to have RVD
had a positive result (false-positive ratio, 0.11). The use of
other criteria or combinations of criteria would yield different

Table 7.1: Proportions of fibromuscular hyperplasia (FM) and arteriosclerosis (AS) in patients with renovascular disease by age and sex.

Age	FM		AS	
	Males	*Females*	*Males*	*Females*
21–40	0.40	0.81	0.60	0.19
41–60	.12	.39	.88	.61

results [Bookstein et al., 1972; McNeil and Adelstein, 1975]. Mortality and morbidity from the IVP were assumed to be negligible, but a mortality rate of 1 per 1,000 during subsequent renal arteriography was assumed, as found in the Cooperative Study [Franklin et al., 1975].

Estimated costs of the diagnostic tests employed were based upon the Massachusetts Relative Value Scale [Interspeciality Committee, 1971]. Rapid-sequence ("hypertensive") intravenous pyelography served as a baseline at $83 per examination. The cost of a renal arteriogram was then computed from the Relative Value Scale to be $375. (This figure excludes the cost of hospitalization usually associated with performing a renal arteriogram and, therefore, underestimates the true cost.) The cost of hospitalization and surgery was estimated on the basis of 1974 charges at the Peter Bent Brigham Hospital to be $5,000 [McNeil et al., 1975].

Assumptions. In addition to estimates of the prevalence of RVD, several assumptions were made regarding the diagnostic strategies employed and the efficacies of surgical and medical treatment.

The net costs and benefits of a lifetime of antihypertensive treatment were drawn from the analyses in chapters 2 and 4. The assumption of incomplete (50 percent) adherence with maximum cost was employed as defined in chapter 4. All costs and benefits were discounted at 5 percent per year although, in a sensitivity analysis, the calculations were repeated without discounting.

In the comparison of surgical and medical management, it was assumed that the blood pressure distributions of patients with and without RVD are similar and that the two groups are at equal risk of fatal or nonfatal complications. Furthermore, it was assumed that surgical survivors subsequently treated medically are at equal risk as medically treated patients.

Medical treatment was assumed to be equally effective in

lowering diastolic blood pressure in all patients, including surgical failures. Nonfatal complications from surgery and the need for a second operation were not considered.

Methods. The cost-effectiveness criterion, as in previous chapters, is the net cost per year of increased quality-adjusted life expectancy (see chapter 2). In this case, the net increase in cost (ΔC) is the expected cost associated with strategy 1 (IVP/surgery) less the expected cost associated with strategy 2 (medical management). The net increase in quality-adjusted life expectancy (ΔE) is similarly defined. The ratio of these is the cost-effectiveness criterion for resource allocation.

Two components of the cost-effectiveness criterion deserve special attention. The first is the expected cost of finding a patient with RVD and effecting a surgical cure. This "cost per surgical cure" (*CPSC*) is defined as follows:

$$CPSC = (C_1 + p_1 C_2 + p_1 p_2 p_3 C_3)/(p_1 p_2 p_3 p_4), \qquad (7.1)$$

where:

C_1	= cost of IVP ($83);
C_2	= cost of arteriography ($375);
C_3	= cost of surgery ($5,000);
p_1	= probability that a screened patient has a positive IVP (0.177);
p_2	= probability that a positive IVP will be confirmed as RVD by arteriography (0.441);
p_3	= probability that a confirmed case of RVD will be operated on (1.0 if FM and AS are operated on) (age-sex-specific rate of FM [table 7.1] if only FM is operated on);
p_4	= surgical cure rate (weighted average of 0.62 for FM, 0.44 for AS [Foster, Maxwell, and Franklin, 1975], the weights being derived from table 7.1);
$p_1 p_2 p_3 p_4$	= probability that a screened patient will be cured surgically.

Values calculated for each age, sex, and surgical substrategy or operability criterion are shown in table 7.2. The *CPSC*s in all cases markedly exceed the present-value lifetime costs of medical therapy, which average an estimated $3,000–$4,000 (chapters 2 and 4), and are higher if only FM is treated surgically. Because

Table 7.2: Cost per surgical cure (*CPSC*) by age, sex, and operability criterion.

Age	Operate on FM only		Operate on FM and AS	
	Males	*Females*	*Males*	*Females*
30	$15,800	$12,000	$13,500	$11,800
50	33,800	16,000	15,000	13,600

women and younger patients have relatively higher proportions of FM, costs per cure are lower than for men and older patients.

The second quantity deserving attention in the cost-effectiveness criterion is the expected number of surgical deaths per cure. The formulation of deaths per surgical cure (*DPSC*) is as follows:

$$DPSC = (p_1 d_2 + p_1 p_2 p_3 d_4)/(p_1 p_2 p_3 p_4), \qquad (7.2)$$

where:

d_2 = mortality rate for arteriography (0.001) [Franklin et al., 1975],

d_4 = mortality rate for surgery (weighted average of 0.034 for FM, 0.093 for AS [Franklin et al., 1975], the weights being derived from table 7.1),

and p_1, p_2, p_3, and p_4 are as defined in equation 7.1. Its computed values by age, sex, and operability criterion are presented in table 7.3. Note that *DPSC* is higher when cases of AS are given surgery because of the higher surgical mortality for AS compared to FM.

Comparison of tables 7.2 and 7.3 highlights the tradeoffs between the decision rules for operability. While operating on FM alone has a higher cost per cure, the mortality rate is significantly lower than if all cases of RVD, including AS, are treated surgically. This tradeoff is also evident in the cost-effectiveness results.

In the cost-effectiveness ratio, $R = \Delta C/\Delta E$, the numerator is the net increase in cost per surgical cure:

$$\Delta C = CPSC - (1 + DPSC) \, \Delta C_{Med}^{Inc \ adh} - \Delta C_{Morb}^{Full \ adh} . \qquad (7.3)$$

This consists of three terms, the first two representing the difference between the gross cost per surgical cure (*CPSC*) and the medical treatment costs that would have been incurred by those who are cured or who die as a result of surgery. (In the equation *DPSC* represents deaths per surgical cure, and $\Delta C_{Med}^{Inc \ adh}$ is defined as the net lifetime costs of medical treatment under

Table 7.3: Deaths per surgical cure (*DPSC*) by age, sex, and operability criterion.

Age	Operate on FM Only		Operate on FM and AS	
	Males	*Females*	*Males*	*Females*
30	0.064	0.059	0.142	0.081
50	.085	.064	.191	.142

incomplete adherence, morbidity and side effects included; see chapter 4.) From this is subtracted the savings in the treatment of subsequent cardiovascular morbid events for those who are cured surgically, whose diastolic blood pressures are lowered to 90 mm Hg. (The term $\Delta C_{Morb}^{Full\ adh}$ equals savings in treatment for cardiovascular morbidity under full adherence.)

The denominator, the net change in quality-adjusted life expectancy per surgical cure, also consists of three terms:

$$\Delta E = \Delta E_{No\ SE}^{Full\ adh} - \Delta E_{With\ SE}^{Inc\ adh} - DPSC\ (LE_{No\ Rx})\ . \qquad (7.4)$$

The first term is the increase in quality-adjusted life expectancy per surgical cure (equivalent to full adherence but without medication side effects). The second, to be subtracted from the first, is the increase in quality-adjusted life expectancy that would be obtained by medical treatment (under incomplete adherence with side effects). The third, also to be subtracted, represents the loss of life due to surgical mortality (where $LE_{No\ Rx}$ is the quality-adjusted life expectancy in the absence of treatment). Equations 7.3 and 7.4 are derived in the appendix to this chapter.

Results. The analysis for individuals with diastolic blood pressures of 110 mm Hg resulted in a net *decrease* in quality-adjusted life expectancy for the IVP/surgery strategy relative to the medical management strategy for both sexes, both age groups, and both criteria for surgery (table 7.4). Thus, unless the IVP/surgery strategy were to show a net *savings* in cost, it would be dominated on both cost and effectiveness grounds by medical management. As shown in the bottom half of table 7.4, however, the IVP/surgery strategy does entail a substantial net increase in cost in all cases. Hence, it can be concluded that it is not cost-effective to screen for renovascular disease, at least under the assumptions used in this analysis.

Although there is both a net loss of health effectiveness and a net increase in cost, it should be noted that the loss of life ex-

Table 7.4: Net effectiveness and cost of the IVP/surgery strategy (strategy 1) relative to the medical management strategy (strategy 2).

Quantity estimated	Age	Operate on FM only		Operate on FM and AS	
		Males	*Females*	*Males*	*Females*
Net change in quality-adjusted life expectancy per surgical cure (years)[a]	30	−0.23	−0.45	−1.39	−0.99
	50	−0.62	−0.43	−1.83	−1.49
Net increase in cost per surgical cure[a]	30	$13,000	$ 9,000	$10,600	$ 8,800
	50	30,400	13,400	12,800	10,900

[a] Discounted at 5% per annum.

pectancy is substantially less when only patients with FM are given surgery although the cost is higher. Moreover, the results are relatively more favorable to the surgical strategy in younger patients. These observations form the basis for the sensitivity analysis.

Discussion and sensitivity analysis. It is important to ascertain the extent to which the strong conclusion against screening for renovascular disease depends on the assumptions made in the model. Since virtually every assumption tends to favor the surgical strategies, however, it is unlikely that realistic changes in these will change the conclusions.

The 10 percent prevalence of RVD is almost certainly an upper bound. While this prevalence might be expected in selected referral populations, it is probably far above that found in community settings. The prevalence of RVD may be expected to vary with age (inversely for the fibromuscular type, and directly for the arteriosclerotic type), but 10 percent is almost surely an upper bound across all ages between 21 and 60. A lower prevalence would make screening even less attractive.

The assumptions of incomplete adherence (50 percent among nondropouts) and maximum cost (chapter 4) put medical management in its worst light. Better adherence would make screening look even worse.

No side effects, nonfatal complications, or need for reoperation was postulated for surgical management. The last assumption was made despite a 14.1 percent reoperation rate in the Cooperative Study [Franklin et al., 1975]. Relaxation of any of these assumptions would further detract from the attractiveness of screening for RVD.

The analysis was limited to persons with diastolic blood pressures of 110 mm Hg. It is not anticipated that the cost-effectiveness of the screening strategy relative to medical management would differ substantially for other blood pressures.

Only two assumptions tended to detract from the screening strategy. One of these was that surgical survivors who are subsequently treated medically are at the same risk as other medically treated patients. This would lead to a slight underestimation of the value of surgery if surgical survivors are actually a lower risk group because of selective operative mortality in high risk patients. It is probable that this effect is not large.

The other assumption, and the only feature of the analysis that appears to warrant formal sensitivity analysis, is the use of discounting of costs and benefits at 5 percent per year. The justification of this procedure was given in chapter 2. Nonetheless, the analysis was repeated without discounting either costs or benefits. Under these circumstances the net effectiveness (ΔE) did turn positive for 30-year-old men and women when only FM led to surgery. Net effectiveness remained negative for 50-year-olds, and for surgery for AS. The net effectiveness remained positive for 30-year-old women when half of such patients with AS were given surgery in addition to those with FM. These results are shown in table 7.5.

To permit computation of cost-effectiveness, the net increase in cost was computed for patient categories in which the net increases in life expectancy became positive (table 7.5). The most favorable ratios are $7,900 and $11,600 per year of increased quality-adjusted life expectancy for 30-year-old women and men, respectively, if only FM is operated upon. Despite the omission of discounting, these ratios still compare very unfavorably to those for medical treatment alone, which are about $4,000 for 30-year-olds (with incomplete adherence). Hence, the IVP/surgery strategy is significantly less cost-effective at the margin than medical treatment alone, and the conclusion of this analysis is further confirmed.

Conclusions

The cost-effectiveness of screening for any known cause of hypertension depends on the prevalence of the condition, the

Table 7.5: Results of sensitivity analysis without discounting, for 30-year-olds.

Quantity estimated	Operate on FM only		Operate on FM and AS		Operate on FM and 1/2 AS[a]	
	Males	*Females*	*Males*	*Females*	*Males*	*Females*
Net change in quality-adjusted life expectancy per surgical cure (years)	+0.85	+0.57	−1.58	−0.28	−0.18	+0.11
Net increase in cost per surgical cure	$ 9,800	$4,500	—	—	—	$ 4,100
Net cost per year of increased quality-adjusted life expectancy	11,600	7,900	—	—	—	39,000

[a] Surgery given to all FM patients and half of AS patients.

presence of identifiable patient characteristics or clinical symptoms that permit targeting of screening, the availability of a reliable screening test and of specific treatment that is significantly more effective than antihypertensive medications alone, and the cost of screening and alternative modes of treatment. All known causes of secondary hypertension are relatively rare in relation to essential hypertension. For conditions that are readily recognized with little or no additional use of resources (coarctation of the aorta, Cushing's disease, contraceptive pill-induced hypertension), no problem arises. When specific treatment is markedly more effective than treatment with antihypertensive medications, and when the cost of delay in establishing the diagnosis may be considerable (possibly the case with pheochromocytoma), the decision to screen is rather clear. The decision becomes more difficult, however, when the diagnostic process is expensive and cost of delay minimal (primary aldosteronism).

For renovascular disease, cost-effectiveness analysis shows that diagnostic evaluation of every hypertensive, followed by surgical treatment for those found to have the disease, is a relatively inefficient use of health resources. This conclusion holds despite the use of assumptions favorable to surgery and rests importantly on both the high cost of a surgical "cure" and the equivocal net effect of surgical treatment on life expectancy. If screening were targeted only at groups of hypertensive patients in which the prevalence of renovascular disease is significantly higher than

10 percent, the analysis would become more favorable toward surgery.

These conclusions, obviously, pertain only to clinical practice and the current state of medical knowledge. Research directed at improving understanding of fundamental mechanisms and developing improved modes of treatment should obviously be judged by very different criteria.

Reasons for the disparity between the current enthusiasm for diagnosing causes of secondary hypertension and the more conservative indications of societal cost-effectiveness are several. First, current health insurance reimbursement programs tend to favor surgical and hospital interventions over ambulatory treatments. A patient treated surgically for renovascular disease may pay virtually nothing out-of-pocket, while a patient following a lifetime course of antihypertensive medications is likely to bear much of the cost. Second, as noted in chapters 4 and 5, medical education tends to emphasize definitive therapy for acute conditions more than long-term or preventive therapy for chronic conditions such as hypertension. Provider satisfaction from achieving a "cure" is likely to exceed that from merely achieving and maintaining blood pressure "control" and its associated unobservable risk reductions. Until these conditions underlying our medical care system change, it is likely that providers will continue to give excessive emphasis to screening for rare, "interesting," and potentially curable forms of hypertension.

Appendix to Chapter 7

The purpose of this appendix is to derive equations 7.3 and 7.4, the numerator and denominator of the cost-effectiveness ratio. Terms used are defined as follows:

p_1 = probability that a screened patient has a positive IVP ($P\{\text{IVP}^+\}$);

p_2 = probability that a positive IVP will be confirmed as RVD by arteriography ($P\{\text{RVD}|\text{IVP}^+\}$);

p_3 = probability that a confirmed case of RVD will be operated upon (either 1.0 or $P\{\text{FM}|\text{RVD}\}$, depending on operability criterion);

p_4 = surgical cure rate ($P\{\text{Cure}|\text{Operate}\}$);

C_1 = cost of IVP;

C_2 = cost of arteriography;

C_3 = cost of surgery;

$CPSC$ = cost per surgical cure (gross) = $(C_1 + p_1 C_2 + p_1 p_2 p_3 C_3)/p_1 p_2 p_3 p_4$;

d_2 = death rate for arteriography;

d_4 = death rate for surgery;

$DPSC$ = deaths per surgical cure = $(p_1 d_2 + p_1 p_2 p_3 d_4)/p_1 p_2 p_3 p_4$;

$\Delta C_{Med}^{Inc\ adh}$ = net lifetime costs of medical treatment under incomplete adherence (morbidity and side effects included; see chapter 4);

$\Delta C_{Morb}^{Full\ adh}$ = savings in treatment of cardiovascular morbidity under full adherence (see chapter 2);

$\Delta E_{No\ SE}^{Full\ adh}$ = increase in quality-adjusted life expectancy for a surgical "cure" (equivalent to full adherence, but without medication side effects; see chapter 2);

215

$\Delta E^{Inc\ adh}_{With\ SE}$ = increase in quality-adjusted life expectancy under incomplete adherence (see chapter 4);

$LE^{Inc\ adh}$ = quality-adjusted life expectancy with treatment and incomplete adherence;

$LE_{No\ Rx}$ = quality-adjusted life expectancy without treatment;

ΔCPP_{Surg} = cost per patient under IVP/surgery strategy;

ΔCPP_{Med} = cost per patient under medical management strategy;

$\Delta LEPP_{Surg}$ = increase in quality-adjusted life expectancy per patient under IVP/surgery strategy;

$\Delta LEPP_{Med}$ = increase in quality-adjusted life expectancy per patient under medical management strategy.

The expected costs per patient under the IVP/surgery strategy include (1) the cost of the IVP, (2) the cost of arteriography for those with positive IVPs, (3) the cost of surgery for those operated upon, and (4) the lifetime cost of medical management for those not cured surgically. From these are subtracted (5) the savings in the costs of treating morbid cardiovascular events for those cured surgically. Thus the expected cost per patient under the IVP/surgery strategy may be written as follows:

$$\Delta CPP_{Surg} = C_1 + p_1 C_2 + p_1 p_2 p_3 C_3$$
$$+ (1 - p_1 p_2 p_3 p_4 - p_1 d_2 - p_1 p_2 p_3 d_4)\ \Delta C^{Inc\ adh}_{Med}$$
$$- p_1 p_2 p_3 p_4\ \Delta C^{Full\ adh}_{Morb}.$$

The expected costs per patient under the medical management strategy are simply:

$$\Delta CPP_{Med} = \Delta C^{Inc\ adh}_{Med}.$$

Combining terms and substituting the definitions of cost per surgical cure ($CPSC$) and deaths per surgical cure ($DPSC$) as given above, the net cost per patient simplifies to:

$$\Delta CPP_{Surg} - \Delta CPP_{Med} = p_1 p_2 p_3 p_4 [CPSC$$
$$- (1 + DPSC)\ \Delta C^{Inc\ adh}_{Med} - \Delta C^{Full\ adh}_{Morb}].$$
$$(7A.1)$$

The expression in brackets in equation 7A.1 may be recognized as equation 7.3, the net increase in cost per surgical cure (ΔC).

The increase in quality-adjusted life expectancy per patient under the IVP/surgery strategy is equal to the weighted average of (1) the increase for those cured surgically, (2) the increase for those not cured surgically but who survive surgery and are treated medically, and (3) the loss of life resulting from the arteriogram or surgery. Thus the expected increase in quality-adjusted life expectancy per patient under the IVP/surgery strategy may be written as:

$$\Delta LEPP_{Surg} = p_1 p_2 p_3 p_4 \, \Delta E^{Full\ adh}_{No\ SE}$$
$$+ (1 - p_1 p_2 p_3 p_4 - p_1 d_2 - p_1 p_2 p_3 d_4) \, \Delta E^{Inc\ adh}_{With\ SE}$$
$$- (p_1 d_2 + p_1 p_2 p_3 d_4) LE^{Inc\ adh}.$$

The increase in quality-adjusted life expectancy per patient under the medical management strategy is simply:

$$\Delta LEPP_{Med} = \Delta E^{Inc\ adh}_{With\ SE} \ .$$

Combining terms and substituting the definition of deaths per surgical cure (*DPSC*) as given above, the net increase in quality-adjusted life expectancy per patient simplifies to:

$$\Delta LEPP_{Surg} - \Delta LEPP_{Med} = p_1 p_2 p_3 p_4 \, [\Delta E^{Full\ adh}_{No\ SE} - \Delta E^{Inc\ adh}_{With\ SE}$$
$$- DPSC \, (LE^{Inc\ adh} - \Delta E^{Inc\ adh})] \ .$$

$$(7A.2)$$

Noting that the difference, $LE^{Inc\ adh} - \Delta E^{Inc\ adh}$, is the baseline life expectancy without treatment, $LE_{No\ Rx}$, the expression in brackets in equation 7A.2 may be recognized as equation 7.4, the net increase in quality-adjusted life expectancy per surgical cure (ΔE).

The cost-effectiveness ratio is the quantity in equation 7A.1 divided by the quantity in equation 7A.2. The term $p_1 p_2 p_3 p_4$, denoting the rate of surgical cures per patient, cancels from both the numerator and the denominator, leaving the expression for $\Delta C / \Delta E$ as defined by equations 7.3 and 7.4.

8. Findings and Recommendations

Because hypertension is one of the most important public health problems in the United States today, it can be argued that a major national effort should be undertaken to ensure that effective treatment is provided to as many untreated or inadequately treated hypertensives as possible. To that end, widespread public screening and intensive education programs at local, state, and national levels have been advocated. But because treatment is costly, is of unproven efficacy in those 70 to 80 percent of hypertensives who have mild elevations in blood pressure, and is frequently accompanied by side effects that may be severe, it can also be argued that better uses could be found for health care dollars. The additional costs required to locate and evaluate individuals who are not currently aware that they have hypertension, and to improve adherence of known hypertensives to lifelong medical regimens, must also be considered.

This analysis of the problem of hypertension is based on the principle that, under conditions of limited resources for health care, society's best interest is served by setting relative priorities for resource use according to the amount of health benefits received per dollar spent. This same principle applies equally well to tradeoffs between hypertension and other health care problems. Moreover, where the tradeoff is between expenditures on health care and on nonhealth programs, any decision implies some valuation of additional health benefits relative to other goods and services that people value. Thus, for example, a decision to increase the national health budget to control hypertension would imply that the health benefits so derived are worth more than the goods and services that could have resulted from alternative uses of those same resources.

The specific policy questions addressed were:

- Should major new resources be devoted to the treatment of hypertension?
- How should priorities for the use of treatment resources be set?
- How should the problem of drug side effects influence treatment and policy decisions?
- Considering that many patients do not adhere to medical regimens, is treatment of hypertension nevertheless a wise use of resources?
- What kinds of public, provider, or patient educational programs should be implemented?
- Should hypertension screening programs be implemented? Under what conditions? For what target populations?
- How should resources be divided among screening, treatment, and follow-up interventions?
- How much effort should be spent in diagnosing the known curable forms of hypertension?
- What incentives can be provided to the patient, the provider, or other decision makers to encourage them to act in the public interest?
- When should action be taken on the basis of incomplete information, and when should the results of further research be awaited? What are the highest priority areas for research?

Principal Findings

CLINICAL TREATMENT OF HYPERTENSION. The annual national cost of treating those with diastolic blood pressures above 105 mm Hg is estimated at $900 million. If, in addition, those with diastolic blood pressures between 95 mm Hg and 105 mm Hg were treated, this annual cost would rise to $2.9 billion. If all adults with diastolic blood pressures above 90 mm Hg were treated, the estimated annual cost would be $4.8 billion.

Medical costs saved by prevention of cardiovascular morbidity in treated hypertensives do not come close to "paying for" the costs of antihypertensive treatment. Only 22 percent of gross treatment costs can be expected to be recovered from savings in the treatment of strokes and heart attacks among those with diastolic blood pressures of 105 mm Hg and above. Therefore, treatment must be justified in terms of the prolongation and improved quality of life it provides, rather than absolute cost savings.

If all persons in the United States with diastolic blood pressures of 105 mm Hg and above were treated, the aggregate net cost per year of increased quality-adjusted life expectancy is estimated to be $4,850, assuming full adherence to therapy. For treatment of persons with diastolic blood pressures from 95 mm Hg to 104 mm Hg, this figure would be $9,880. Hence, treatment of "mild" hypertension (95 to 104 mm Hg), even if it were proven to be effective, would be more than twice as costly as that of moderate and severe hypertension ($\geq$ 105 mm Hg) per unit of health benefit achieved and, hence, may not be a cost-effective use of health resources.

Cost-effectiveness considerations result in priorities for treatment by blood pressure level, age, and sex (figures 2.13 and 2.14). It appears to be more cost-effective to treat higher blood pressures, younger men, and older women (figures 2.11 and 2.12). The potential value of initiating treatment early in life for men is particularly impressive. Better data are urgently needed to verify the effectiveness of treatment in young people.

Estimates of cost-effectiveness are sensitive to the extent to which blood pressure control eliminates the excess risk associated with the pretreatment blood pressure level. Cost-effectiveness under various assumptions about this "fraction of benefit" is shown in figures 2.6 and 2.7. Available empirical studies do not adequately deal with this fundamental quantitative question.

The dollar cost of antihypertensive medications is of great importance in determining cost-effectiveness, since such medications are taken throughout the patient's lifetime. Differences in cost among commonly used drug regimens, and between generic and proprietary drugs, are, therefore, of major importance. A reduction of drug costs by half improves the cost-effectiveness of treatment by about one-third.

Finally, the mild, chronic, and often subjective side effects of antihypertensive medications may substantially diminish the net effectiveness of treatment by their adverse effects on the quality of life. Benefits of treatment may be reduced by 20 to 50 percent or more, depending on patients' attitudes and preferences regarding these side effects. The impact is especially striking for the treatment of mild hypertension, where benefits, if present, are relatively small.

SIDE EFFECTS OF TREATMENT.   The potential impact of reserpine-induced breast cancer on the cost-effectiveness of treating mild and moderate hypertension in women is substantial. Further studies are needed to resolve uncertainties about this association. The cost-effectiveness of reserpine use is also moderately sensitive to assumptions concerning the incidence and effects of depression, particularly in males. With these exceptions, the impact on cost-effectiveness of mortality and increased medical costs due to known side effects of reserpine, methyldopa, and thiazide diuretics is small. Subjective side effects that impair the quality of life are almost certainly more important than these objective ones.

OBSTACLES TO EFFECTIVE BLOOD PRESSURE CONTROL. The problem of incomplete adherence to antihypertensive regimens has a substantial adverse effect on the cost-effectiveness of antihypertensive therapy (figures 4.1 and 4.2). If treatment were provided to all persons in the United States with diastolic blood pressures 105 mm Hg or above, the average cost per year of increased quality-adjusted life expectancy could easily be as high as $10,500, compared to $4,850 under full adherence. For treatment of persons with diastolic blood pressures of 95 mm Hg to 104 mm Hg, these figures range as high as $20,400, compared to $9,880 under full adherence. Thus, the anticipation of incomplete adherence may dictate against treatment for many classes of patients, particularly mild hypertensives.

Interventions to improve adherence are generally of unproven efficacy. If even moderate effectiveness can be established, however, treatment supplemented by such interventions would be more cost-effective than treatment alone under most reasonable assumptions regarding the costs of such interventions (figure 4.3).

The role of the provider in relation to the adherence problem has been generally underemphasized. Greater attention in medical education to the management of chronic, asymptomatic health problems such as hypertension and efforts to heighten provider awareness of the adherence problem and of the importance of patient–provider communication are avenues deserving further exploration. Increased utilization of specially trained allied health personnel also shows promise.

Patient education is another approach to the adherence problem that has been advocated. Evidence suggests that, to be effective, it needs to be coupled with behavioral reinforcement. The use of tangible rewards (for example, monetary incentives) is theoretically appealing in this regard.

SCREENING FOR HYPERTENSION.   Problems with patient adherence, failure of providers to initiate therapy, and failure of screening programs to refer patients successfully to medical care, all severely compromise the cost-effectiveness of widespread public screening for hypertension. The present-value cost of a screening program applied to the entire United States adult population would be about $1.1 billion, plus the costs of diagnostic evaluation, treatment, and follow-up. Its estimated net cost per year of quality-adjusted life expectancy ranges from $6,600 under full adherence, to between $11,400 and $15,500 under various assumptions made regarding incomplete adherence (table 5.5). Screening coupled with efforts to improve subsequent adherence is substantially more cost-effective than screening alone, even if the interventions have high unit costs and are of only moderate effectiveness (table 5.5).

If screening is to be done, and resources are limited, referral for treatment should be limited to those with moderate and severe hypertension, and blood pressure cutoff levels should vary with age and sex. This is not meant to imply that individuals with lower blood pressures should be ignored; they should be urged to remain under medical surveillance.

Screening in selected target populations, notably black populations, is likely to be more cost-effective than community-wide screening, provided that subsequent adherence is no worse than in the general population (table 5.5). Targeting by age, however, is not particularly cost-effective.

Screening at sources of regular medical care is likely to be more cost-effective than mass public screening due to the elimination of attrition in referral. Estimates of the net cost per year of increased quality-adjusted life expectancy range from $8,400 to $12,000 under different adherence assumptions (table 5.5). The success of the "private" approach depends importantly, however, on the criteria providers use to initiate treatment in hypertensives, and on the efforts they make to encourage adherence. Moreover, total reliance on private screening will result in the exclusion of individuals who are isolated from the health care system.

RESOURCE ALLOCATION IN COMMUNITY HYPERTENSION PROGRAMS.   A program with limited resources will maximize total health benefits by concentrating its efforts on proadherence interventions, even at a sacrifice in terms of the numbers screened and treated. This conclusion holds even if such interventions are very expensive and only moderately effective, and even if screening is very inexpensive.

DIAGNOSIS AND TREATMENT OF SECONDARY HYPERTENSION. The cost-effectiveness of extensive screening and diagnostic evaluation for secondary causes of hypertension is dubious. For renovascular disease, the most common of the surgically curable causes of hypertension, analysis reveals that medical antihypertensive treatment is, in general, considerably more cost-effective.

Recommendations

The diffuse nature of the health care system, with its multiplicity of institutions, providers, suppliers, regulatory bodies, and sources of financing, makes the implementation of change in health policies an extremely complex matter. Different decision makers have different objectives and respond to different incentives. Hence no set of recommendations will be attractive to all, and no simple set of actions will uniformly result in the desired outcomes. Implementation of cost-effective policies will be facilitated greatly by institutional changes such as quality assurance and utilization control programs, prepayment mechanisms, and national health insurance. The following recommendations that result from this analysis are made with the realization that multiple factors may shape their implementation.

Criteria for allocating treatment resources cost-effectively among various patient groups should be disseminated to and reinforced by fiscal intermediaries, prepaid health plans, regulatory agencies, and peer review groups. It is suggested that: (a) treatment decisions be based on age- and sex-specific blood pressure cutoff levels derived from cost-effectiveness criteria, rather than on arbitrary definitions of "hypertension" or on cutoff levels derived from the distribution of blood pressures in the population; (b) priority for treatment be given to younger men and older women; (c) careful monitoring of subjective side effects of medications be performed routinely and explicitly with subsequent adjustment of dosage and agent, as indicated; and (d) major attention be given to follow-up and efforts to ensure adherence. Curricula of pre- and post-doctoral programs in medical education should take these principles into account.

Major efforts should be undertaken to develop a portfolio of strategies to improve patient adherence, including better access to care, patient education and provider education, and provision of incentives for patient adherence. Development of such methods should be the goal of every provider and health care institution. Evaluation should be conducted through organized research efforts sponsored by the National Institutes of Health and its National High Blood Pressure Education Program, and by other governmental or private organizations with interest in improved health care. Such efforts would have obvious implications for the management of many health care problems beyond hypertension.

Mechanisms should be established to provide financial reimbursement for services that incorporate efforts, by validated methods, to improve adherence. Fiscal intermediaries, including national health insurance and prepaid health care programs, should include such provisions.

Large-scale public programs to detect and treat hypertension are not indicated, at the present time, on the basis of cost-effectiveness considerations. Community hypertension programs and their sponsors should, therefore, allocate resources to proadherence activities in preference to widespread screening efforts.

Public screening programs in black communities are substantially more cost-effective than community-wide screening because of the extraordinarily high prevalence and severity of hypertension in blacks. Implementation is recommended, provided that resources for ensuring treatment and follow-up are available.

Screening for hypertension during health care encounters for other purposes is more cost-effective than public screening and should be encouraged, especially for primary care providers. Implementation of this recommendation might reasonably involve medical educational institutions and professional groups as well as fiscal intermediaries. The use of financial incentives to reward providers for screening that results in subsequent control of hypertension should be explored.

Less incentive should be given to providers to conduct elaborate and expensive diagnostic workups for secondary causes of hypertension and more incentive for detecting and effectively treating patients with essential hypertension. Such incentives could be provided by fiscal intermediaries by changing existing reimbursement policies that favor surgery, by quality assurance programs, and by prepaid health care plans.

The use of generic drugs should be encouraged to lower the cost of antihypertensive treatment.

Resources should be expended to permit both the National Institutes of Health and the pharmaceutical industry to develop antihypertensive medications that not only are more effective in lowering blood pressure but also are less costly to produce and less likely to cause side effects at required dosages.

Priorities in hypertension research should be based on resolving those uncertainties concerning the magnitude of the benefits and risks of antihypertensive treatment that bear most heavily on cost-effectiveness. Areas of priority include: (a) determination of the relationship between blood pressure elevations in childhood and subsequent excess risk, and of the benefits of early detection and treatment; (b) determination of the extent of the benefit of treatment relative to full elimination of excess risk, especially for mild and moderate hypertension; (c) determination of the prevalence of, and patient attitudes toward, subjective side effects of medication; and (d) demonstration and evaluation of alternative methods to improve patient adherence to antihypertensive regimens.

The Analysis in Perspective

Limitations of this analysis that bear upon its findings, its recommendations, and their possible implementation need to be acknowledged.

First, the information upon which the analysis was based is imperfect. Estimates of mortality and morbidity were derived from a single prospective cohort study, the Framingham Heart Study. In our opinion, this represents the best available data source. Nonetheless, both the statistical reliability of its findings and their applicability to the United States population at large are open to question. Other data relating to hypertension were drawn from the medical literature. Where the information needed was incomplete, subjective estimates were supplied; where it was totally lacking, alternative assumptions covering the spectrum of possibilities were tested. Clearly, new data should be incorporated into the structure of this analysis as they become available. As we have stressed from the outset, however, current decisions do have to be made and frequently cannot await the availability of conclusive information.

Second, it should be emphasized that the viewpoint represented throughout is that of the public, of society. Each policy maker, administrator, health care provider, and patient will have his own objectives, biases, and constraints. Each will, and should, interpret our findings accordingly to arrive at his own conclusions for his own decision-making purposes.

Finally, we must acknowledge the ethical issues that arise when considering recommendations concerning public programs and public policies to improve health. It can be argued that public screening and efforts to ensure adherence, while they may operate to the public good, also may constitute infringements on human rights, interfering with the rights of individuals to spend their money and promote their health as they wish. Such dilemmas and their resolution are not within the scope of this analysis. They should, however, be kept in mind while evaluating it.

Policy change requires a long-term commitment. The conclusions and recommendations reached by this analysis apply only to today's decisions about hypertension, in the present institutional environment, with the current information base. As we learn more about the causes of hypertension, preventive measures applied through changes in lifestyle and diet, or curative measures developed through basic research, may diminish the need for drug therapy, thus raising very different issues for screening and management of the condition. Likewise, changes in health care institutions and their financing mechanisms will undoubtedly occur, both creating new opportunities and incentives for decision makers to adopt desirable practices toward hypertension, and raising some new barriers and disincentives in the process. Moreover, while this analysis focuses on hypertension as a categorical health problem, the management of this condition cannot be clearly separated from that of other health problems or from the structure of the health care system within which all services are provided. The challenge is to refine the structural framework of the analysis, broaden its application to other health problems, and keep its continuously updated results before us as a guide to future policy decisions.

Bibliography
Index

Bibliography

Acton, J. P. 1973. *Evaluating Public Programs to Save Lives: The Case of Heart Attacks.* Report R950 RC. Santa Monica: The Rand Corporation.

Alderman, M. H., and Schoenbaum, E. E. 1975. Detection and treatment of hypertension at the worksite. *N. Engl. J. Med.* 293: 65–68.

American Heart Association. 1974. *High Blood Pressure Control: A Guide for Community Programs.* Prepared by the Sub-Committee of Reduction of Risk of Heart Attack and Stroke. New York: American Heart Association.

Armstrong, B.; Stevens, N.; and Doll, R. 1974. Retrospective study of the association between the use of Rauwolfia derivatives and breast cancer in English women. *Lancet* 2:672–675.

Aronow, W. S.; Allen, W. H.; and De Cristofaro, D. 1975. Response of patients and physicians to mass screening for coronary risk factors. *Circulation* 52:586–588.

Ayers, C. R.; Slaughter, A. R.; Smallwood, H. D.; Taylor, F. E.; and Weitzman, R. E. 1973. Standards for quality care of hypertensive patients in office and hospital practice. *Am. J. Cardiol.* 32:533–545.

Bachrach, W. H. 1959. Reserpine, gastric secretion and peptic ulcer. *Am. J. Dig. Dis.* 4:117–124.

Becker, M. H., and Maiman, L. A. 1975. Sociobehavioral determinants of compliance with health and medical care recommendations. *Med. Care* 13:10–24.

Benson, H.; Rosner, B. A.; Marzetta, B. R.; and Klemchuk, H. M. 1974. Decreased blood pressure in pharmacologically treated hypertensive patients who regularly elicited the relaxation response. *Lancet* 1:289–291.

Berg, R. L. 1973. Establishing the values of various conditions of life for a health status index. In *Health Status Indexes: Proceedings of a Conference Conducted by Health Services Research, Tucson, Arizona, 1972,* ed. R. L. Berg. Chicago: Hospital Research and Educational Trust.

Berger, L., and Yu, T. F. 1975. Renal function in gout. *Am. J. Med.* 59:605–613.

Bernstein, S., and Kaufman, M. R. 1960. A psychological analysis of apparent depression following Rauwolfia therapy. *J. Mt. Sinai Hosp.* 27:525–530.

Bjork, S.; Sannerstedt, R.; Falkheden, T.; and Hood, B. 1961. The effect of active drug treatment in severe hypertensive disease. *Acta Med. Scand.* 169:673–689.

Blackwell, B. 1973. Patient compliance. *N. Engl. J. Med.* 289:249–252.

Blood, J. 1974. Housewares a premium winner for buyers at Chicago show. *Merchandising Weekly* 8 October, p. 18.

————. 1973. Sales incentives—fastest growing use of premiums. *Merchandising Weekly* 28 October, p. 1.

Bookstein, J. J.; Abrams, H. L.; Buenger, R. E.; Lecky, J.; Franklin, S. S.; Reiss, M. D.; Bleifer, K. H.; Klatte, E. C.; Varady, P. D.; and Maxwell, M. H. 1972. Radiologic aspects of renovascular hypertension. *J.A.M.A.* 220:1225–1230.

Borhani, N. O. 1975. Implementation and evaluation of community hypertension programs. In *Epidemiology and Control of Hypertension,* ed. O. Paul. New York: Stratton Intercontinental Medical Book Corporation.

Borhani, N. O., and Borkman, J. S. 1968. *Alameda County Blood Pressure Study.* Berkeley: State of California Department of Public Health.

Boston Collaborative Drug Surveillance Program. 1974. Reserpine and breast cancer. *Lancet* 2:672–675.

Bötliger, L. E., and Westerholm, B. 1973. Acquired haemolytic anaemia. Part 2: Drug-induced haemolitic anaemia. *Acta Med. Scand.* 193:227–231.

Brook, R. H., and Appel, F. A. 1973. Quality-of-care assessment: choosing a method for peer review. *N. Engl. J. Med.* 288:1323–1329.

Bryant, J. M.; Yu, T. F.; Berger, L.; Schvartz, N.; Torosdag, S.; Fletcher, L.; Fertig, H.; Schwartz, M. S.; and Quan, R. B. F. 1962. Hyperuricemia induced by the administration of chlorthalidone and other sulfonamide diuretics. *Am. J. Med.* 33:408–420.

Bulpitt, C. J., and Dollery, C. T. 1973. Side effects of hypotensive agents evaluated by a self-administered questionnaire. *Br. Med. J.* 2:485–490.

Bush, J. W.; Chen, M. M.; and Patrick, D. L. 1973. Health status index in cost-effectiveness: analysis of PKU program. In *Health Status Indexes: Proceedings of a Conference Conducted by Health Services Research, Tucson, Arizona, 1972,* ed. R. L. Berg. Chicago: Hospital Research and Educational Trust.

Caldwell, J. R.; Cobb, S.; Dowling, M. D.; and de Jongh, D. 1970. The dropout problem in antihypertensive treatment. *J. Chronic Dis.* 22:579–592.

Carstairs, K. C.; Breckenridge, A.; Dollery, C. T.; and Worlledge, S. M.

1966. Incidence of a positive direct Coombs test in patients on alpha-methyldopa. *Lancet* 2:133–135.

Center for Disease Control. 1975a. (United States Department of Health, Education, and Welfare, Public Health Service.) *Morbidity and Mortality* 24(19):165–166. Atlanta.

Center for Disease Control. 1975b. (United States Department of Health, Education, and Welfare, Public Health Service.) *Morbidity and Mortality* 24(30):259–260. Atlanta.

Charman, R. C. 1974. Hypertension management program in an industrial community. *J.A.M.A.* 227:287–291.

Colwill, J. M.; Dutton, A. M.; Morrissey, J.; and Yu, P. N. 1964. Alpha-methyldopa and hydrochlorothiazide. *N. Engl. J. Med.* 271:696–703.

Curry, P. J.; Haskell, W. L.; Stern, M. P.; and Farquhar, J. W. 1976. Results of a two-year health education campaign on systolic blood pressure (sbp): Stanford Three Community Study. *CVD Epidemiology Newsletter* (Council on Epidemiology, American Heart Association) January, p. 48.

Dawber, T. R.; Meadors, G. F.; and Moore, F. E., Jr. 1951. Epidemiological approaches to heart disease: the Framingham Study. *Am. J. Pub. Health* 41:279–286.

Dinon, L. R.; Kim, Y. S.; and Vander Veer, J. B. 1958. Clinical experience with chlorothiazide (Diuril) with particular emphasis on untoward responses: a report of 121 cases studied over a 15-month period. *Am. J. Med. Sci.* 236:533–545.

Dollery, C. T. 1965. Methyldopa in the treatment of hypertension. *Prog. Cardiovasc. Dis.* 8:278–289.

Drug Topics Red Book, 1975. Oradell, New Jersey: Medical Economics Company.

Dustan, H. P.; Schneckloth, R. E.; Corcoran, A. C.; and Page, I. H. 1958. The effectiveness of long term treatment of malignant hypertension. *Circulation* 18:644–651.

Edmonds, C. J., and Jasani, B. 1972. Total body potassium in hypertensive patients during prolonged diuretic therapy. *Lancet* 2:8–12.

Elkington, S. G.; Schreiber, W. M.; and Conn, H. O. 1969. Hepatic injury caused by L-alpha-methyldopa. *Circulation* 40:589–595.

Emlet, H. E., Jr.; Williamson, J. W.; Dittmer, D. L.; and Davis, J. L. 1973. *Estimated Health Benefits and Costs of Post-Onset Care for Stroke.* Analytic Services, Inc. (ANSER); Johns Hopkins University; Interstudy, American Rehabilitation Foundation. Falls Church, Va.: ANSER.

Epstein, F. H.; Ostrander, L. D., Jr.; and Johnson, B. C. 1965. Epidemiological studies of cardiovascular disease in a total community—Tecumseh, Michigan. *Ann. Intern. Med.* 72:1170–1187.

Fanshel, S., and Bush, J. W. 1970. A health status index and its application to health-services outcomes. *Operations Research* 18:1021–1066.

Feinleib, M. 1974. Personal communication.

Feinleib, M.; Garrison, R.; Borhani, N.; Rosenman, R.; and Christian, J. 1975. Studies of hypertension in twins. In *Epidemiology and Control of Hypertension,* ed. O. Paul. New York: Stratton Intercontinental Medical Book Corporation.

Finnerty, F. A., Jr.; Mattie, E. C.; and Finnerty, F. A., III. 1973. Hypertension in the inner city. Part 1: Analysis of clinic drop-outs. *Circulation* 47:73–75.

Finnerty, F. A., Jr.; Shaw, L. W.; and Himmelsbach, C. K. 1973. Hypertension in the inner city. Part 2: Detection and follow-up. *Circulation* 47:76–78.

Forst, B. E. 1973. Quantifying the patient's preference. In *Health Status Indexes: Proceedings of a Conference Conducted by Health Services Research, Tucson, Arizona, 1972,* ed. R. L. Berg. Chicago: Hospital Research and Educational Trust.

Foster, S. H.; Maxwell, M. H.; and Franklin, S. S. 1975. Renovascular occlusive disease: results of operative treatment. *J.A.M.A.* 231:1043–1048.

Franklin, S. S.; Young, J. D.; Maxwell, M. H.; Foster, J. H.; Palmer, J. M.; Cerny, J.; and Varady, P. D. 1975. Operative morbidity and mortality in renovascular disease. *J.A.M.A.* 231:1148–1153.

Frohlich, E. D.; Emmott, C.; Hammarsten, J. E.; Linehan, W. M.; Pollack, D.; and Horseley, A. W. 1971. Evaluation of the initial care of hypertensive patients. *J.A.M.A.* 218:1036–1038.

Gifford, R. W., Jr. 1969. Evaluation of the hypertensive patient with emphasis on detecting curable causes. *Milbank Mem. Fund Q.* 47:170–186.

Glontz, G. E., and Saslaw, S. 1968. Methyldopa fever. *Arch. Intern. Med.* 122:445–447.

Goodwin, F. K.; Ebert, M. H.; and Bunney, W. E., Jr. 1972. Mental effects of reserpine in man: a review. In *Psychiatric Complications of Medical Drugs,* ed. R. I. Shader. New York: Raven Press.

Green, L. W. 1974. Toward cost-benefit evaluations of health education: some concepts, methods, and examples. *Health Education Monographs* 2(3) supplement 1.

Gutmann, M. C., and Benson, H. 1971. Interaction of environmental factors and systemic arterial blood pressure: a review. *Medicine* 50:543–553.

Haagensen, C. D. 1971. *Diseases of the Breast.* 2nd ed. Philadelphia: Saunders.

Hall, A. P.; Barry, P. E.; Dawber, T. R.; and McNamara, P. M. 1967. Epidemiology of gout and hyperuricemia. *Am. J. Med.* 42:27–37.

Hamilton, M. 1966. Selection of patients for antihypertensive therapy. In *Antihypertensive Therapy: Principles and Practice, an International Symposium,* ed. F. Gross. New York: Springer Verlag.

Harrington, M.; Kincaid-Smith, P.; and McMichael, J. 1959. Results of treatment in malignant hypertension. *Brit. Med. J.* 2:969–980.

Harris, Louis and Associates, Inc. 1973. (United States Department of Health, Education, and Welfare.) *The Public and High Blood Pressure.* Survey conducted for the National Heart and Lung Institute. DHEW publication no. (NIH) 74–356. Bethesda, Maryland.

Haskell, W. L.; Stern, M. P.; Wood, P. D.; Brown, W. B.; Farquhar, J. W.; and Maccoby, N. 1974. A multifactor education campaign to reduce cardiovascular risk in three communities: physiological results. *Circulation* 50(4) supplement 3:III–101.

Haynes, R. B., and Sackett, D. L. 1974. *An Annotated Bibliography on the Compliance of Patients with Therapeutic Regimens.* Hamilton, Ontario: McMaster University Medical School.

Health Resources Administration. 1973. (United States Department of Health, Education, and Welfare.) *Expenditures for Personal Health Services: National Trends and Variations 1953–1970,* Ronald Andersen, study director. DHEW publication no. (HRA) 74–3105. Rockville, Maryland.

Heinonen, O. P.; Shapiro, S.; Tuominen, L.; and Turunen, M. I. 1974. Reserpine use in relation to breast cancer. *Lancet* 2: 675–677.

Henry, J. P., and Cassel, J. C. 1969. Psychological factors in essential hypertension. *Am. J. Epidemiol.* 90:171–200.

Horwitz, D.; Pettinger, W. A.; Orvis, H.; Thomas, R. E.; and Sjoerdsma, A. 1967. Effects of methyldopa in fifty hypertensive patients. *Clin. Pharmacol. Ther.* 8:224–234.

Horwitz, N. 1976. Post-op patients forget, fabricate, even deny having consent talks. *Medical Tribune* 25 February, p. 1.

Howard, R. A. 1968. Decision analysis: applied decision theory. In *Proceedings of the Fourth International Conference on Operations Research, 1966,* ed. D. B. Hertz and J. Melese. New York: Wiley.

Interspecialty Committee. 1971. *Special Services and Billing Procedures, Massachusetts Relative Value Study, 1971.* Boston: Massachusetts Medical Society.

Inui, T. S. 1973. Effects of post-graduate physician education on the management and outcomes of patients with hypertension.

Master's thesis, Johns Hopkins University, School of Hygiene and Public Health.

Johnson, P.; Kitchin, A. H.; Lowther, C. P.; and Turner, R. W. D. 1966. Treatment of hypertension with methyldopa. *Br. Med. J.* 1:133–137.

Jones, S. H.; Carr, J.; Hauck, W. W., Jr.; Peterson, O. L.; Colton, T.; and Nickerson, R. J. 1975. Medicare impact of hospital utilization and financing. Unpublished report, Department of Preventive and Social Medicine, Harvard Medical School.

Joyce, C. R. B.; Caple, G.; Mason, M.; Reynolds, E., and Mathews, J. A. 1969. Quantitative study of doctor-patient communication. *Q.J. Med.* 38:183–194.

Kannel, W. B., and Gordon, T., eds. 1970. *The Framingham Study: An Epidemiological Investigation of Cardiovascular Disease,* section 26. Washington, D.C.: Government Printing Office, December.

————. 1974. *The Framingham Study: An Epidemiological Investigation of Cardiovascular Disease,* section 30. DHEW publication no. (NIH) 74–599. Washington, D.C.: Government Printing Office.

Kaplan, N. M. 1973. *Clinical Hypertension.* New York: Medcom Press.

Katz, R. C., and Zlutnick, S. 1975. *Behavior Therapy and Health Care: Principles and Applications.* New York: Pergamon Press.

Kazdin, A. E. 1975. Recent advances in token economy research. In *Progress in Behavior Modification,* ed. W. Hersen; R. Eisler; and P. Miller. New York: Academic Press.

Klarman, H. E. 1965. Syphilis control programs. In *Measuring the Benefits of Government Investments,* ed. R. Dorfman. Washington: The Brookings Institution.

Klein, H. O., and Kaminsky, N. 1973. Methyldopa fever. *N.Y. State J. Med.* 73:448–451.

Knudsen, K. D.; Iwai, J.; and Dahl, L. K. 1973. Salt, heredity and hypertension. In *Hypertension: Mechanisms and Management: The Twenty-Sixth Hahnemann Symposium,* ed. G. Onesti. New York: Grune and Stratton.

Kohner, E. M.; Dollery, C. T.; Lowry, C.; and Schumer, B. 1971. Effect of diuretic therapy on glucose tolerance in hypertensive patients. *Lancet* 1:986-990.

Komaroff, A. L.; Black, W. L.; Flatley, M.; Knopp, R. H.; Reiffen, B.; and Sherman, H. 1974. Protocols for physician assistants: management of diabetes and hypertension. *N. Engl. J. Med.* 290:307-312.

Kramer, M.; Pollack, E. S.; Redick, R. W.; and Locke, B. Z. 1972. *Mental Disorders/Suicide.* Cambridge: Harvard University Press.

Langfeld, S. B. 1973. Hypertension: deficient care of the medically served. *Ann. Intern. Med.* 78:19–23.

Laragh, J. H. 1972. Evaluation and care of the hypertensive patient. *Am. J. Med.* 52:565–569.

Laska, E. M.; Siegel, C.; Meisner, M.; Fischer, S.; and Wanderling, J. 1975. Matched-pairs study of reserpine use and breast cancer. *Lancet* 2:296–300.

Leemhuis, M. P., and Struyvenberg, A. 1973. Significance of hypokalaemia due to diuretics. *Neth. J. Med.* 16:18–28.

Levine, R. J., and Landsberg, L. 1974. Catecholamines and the adrenal medulla. In *Duncan's Diseases of Metabolism*, ed. P. K. Bondy and L. E. Rosenberg. 7th ed. Philadelphia: Saunders.

Lew, E. A. 1973. High blood pressure, other risk factors and longevity: the insurance viewpoint. *Am. J. Med.* 55:281–294.

Lewis, C. E., and Resnik, B. A. 1967. Nurse clinics and progressive ambulatory patient care. *N. Engl. J. Med.* 277:1236–1241.

Ley, P., and Spelman, M. S. 1965. Communications in an outpatient setting. *Br. J. Soc. Clin. Psychol.* 4:114–116.

Mack, T. M.; Henderson, B. E.; Gerkins, V. R.; Arthur, M.; Baptista, J.; and Pike, M. C. 1975. Reserpine and breast cancer in a retirement community. *N. Engl. J. Med.* 292:1366–1371.

Mann, G. V. 1974. The influence of obesity on health. Part 2. *N. Engl. J. Med.* 291:226–232.

Manner, R. J.; Brechbill, D. O.; and Dewitt, K. 1972. Prevalence of hypokalemia in diuretic therapy. *Clin. Med.* 79:15–18.

Maxwell, M. H.; Bleifer, K. H.; Franklin, S. S.; and Varady, P. D. 1972. Demographic analysis of the study. *J.A.M.A.* 220:1195–1204.

McKenney, J. M. 1974. Antihypertensive drug therapy. *J. Am. Pharm. Assoc.* 14:204–212+.

McKenney, J. M.; Slining, J. M.; Henderson, H. R.; Devins, D.; and Barr, M. 1973. The effect of clinical pharmacy services on patients with essential hypertension. *Circulation* 48:1104–1111.

McKeown, T. 1968. Validation of screening procedures. In *Screening in Medical Care*, ed. T. McKeown. London: Oxford University Press.

McNeil, B. J., and Adelstein, S. J. 1975. The value of case finding in hypertensive renovascular disease. *N. Engl. J. Med.* 293:221–226.

McNeil, B. J.; Varady, P. D.; Burrows, B. A.; and Adelstein, S. J. 1975. Cost-effectiveness in hypertensive renovascular diseases. *N. Engl. J. Med.* 293:216–221.

Miall, W. E., and Chinn, S. 1974. Screening for hypertension: some epidemiological observations. *Br. Med. J.* 3:595–600.

Miall, W. E., and Oldham, P. D. 1958. Factors influencing blood pressure in the general population. *Clin. Sci.* 17:409–444.

Miller, G. E. 1967. Continuing education for what? *J. Med. Educ.* 42:320–326.

Mohler, E. R., and Freis, E. D. 1960. Five-year survival of patients with malignant hypertension treated with antihypertensive agents. *Am. Heart J.* 60:329–335.

National Center for Health Statistics. 1973a. (United States Department of Health, Education, and Welfare.) *Current Estimates from the Health Interview Survey: United States—1971.* Vital and Health Statistics, series 10, no. 79. DHEW publication no. (HSM) 73-1505. Washington, D.C.: Government Printing Office.

National Center for Health Statistics. 1973b. (United States Department of Health, Education, and Welfare.) *Prevalence of Selected Chronic Digestive Conditions, United States, July–December 1968.* Vital and Health Statistics, series 10, no. 83. Washington, D.C.: Government Printing Office.

National Center for Health Statistics. 1968. (United States Department of Health, Education, and Welfare.) *United States Life Tables 1959–61,* vol. 1, no. 3. pp. 4–11. Public Health Service publication no. 1252 (vol. 1, nos. 1–6). Washington, D.C.: Public Health Service, June.

National Center for Health Statistics. 1964a. (United States Department of Health, Education, and Welfare.) *Blood Pressure of Adults by Age and* Sex. Vital and Health Statistics, series 11, no. 4. Washington, D.C.: Government Printing Office.

National Center for Health Statistics. 1964b. (United States Department of Health, Education, and Welfare.) *Blood Pressure of Adults by Race and Area. United States—1960–1962.* Vital and Health Statistics, series 11, no. 5. Washington, D.C.: Government Printing Office.

National Heart and Lung Institute. 1974. (United States Department of Health, Education, and Welfare.) *The Underwriting Significance of Hypertension for the Life Insurance Industry.* Prepared for the National High Blood Pressure Education Program. DHEW publication no. (NIH) 74-426. Bethesda, Maryland.

National High Blood Pressure Education Program. 1975. Education of physicians in high blood pressure: performance characteristics, learning objectives and evaluation approaches. *Circulation* 51 (May: News from the American Heart Association): 9–27.

National High Blood Pressure Education Program. 1974. (United States Department of Health, Education, and Welfare.) *National High Blood Pressure Education Program Fact Sheet.* National Heart and Lung Institute, National Institutes of Health. Bethesda, Maryland.

National High Blood Pressure Education Program. 1973a. (United States Department of Health, Education, and Welfare.) *Executive Summary of the Task Force Reports to the Hypertension Information and Education Advisory Committee.* DHEW publication no. (NIH) 74-592. Bethesda, Maryland.

National High Blood Pressure Education Program. 1973b. (United States Department of Health, Education, and Welfare.) *Report to the Hypertension Information and Education Advisory Committee, Task Force I: Data Base.* DHEW publication no. (NIH) 74-593. Bethesda, Maryland.

National High Blood Pressure Education Program. 1973c. (United States Department of Health, Education, and Welfare.) *Report to the Hypertension Information and Education Advisory Committee, Task Force II: Professional Education.* DHEW publication no. (NIH) 74-594. Bethesda, Maryland.

National High Blood Pressure Education Program. 1973d. (United States Department of Health, Education, and Welfare.) *Report to the Hypertension Information and Education Advisory Committee, Task Force III: Community Education.* DHEW publication no. (NIH) 74-595. Bethesda, Maryland.

National High Blood Pressure Education Program. 1973e. (United States Department of Health, Education, and Welfare.) *Report to the Hypertension Information and Education Advisory Committee, Task Force IV: Resource and Impact Assessment.* DHEW publication no. (NIH) 74-596. Bethesda, Maryland.

Newman, R. J., and Salerno, H. R. 1974. Sexual dysfunction due to methyldopa. *Br. Med. J.* 4:106.

Oberman, A.; Castle, C. N.; Daugherty, S.; Detels, R.; Hawkins, C. M.; Krishan, J.; and Wassertreil-Smoller, S. 1974. Results of a two stage screen for hypertension in 14 communities. Unpublished report presented at the American Heart Association National Meeting, Dallas, Texas, 20 November.

O'Fallon, W. M.; Labarthe, D. R.; and Kurland, L. T. 1975. Rauwolfia derivatives and breast cancer. *Lancet* 2:292–296.

Opfell, R. W. 1973. The role of state medical associations in continuing medical education. *J.A.M.A.* 225:732.

Opsahl, R. L., and Dunnette, M. D. 1966. The role of financial compensation in industrial motivation. *Psychol. Bull.* 66:94–118.

Page, L. B.; Damon, A.; and Moellering, R. C. 1974. Antecedents of cardiovascular disease in six Solomon Islands societies. *Circulation* 49:1132–1146.

Parker, W. A. 1974. Methyldopa hyperpyrexia. *J.A.M.A.* 228:1097.

Parsons, H. M. 1974. What happened at Hawthorne? *Science* 183: 922–932.

Patel, C., and North, W. R. S. 1975. Randomized controlled trial of yoga and bio-feedback in management of hypertension. *Lancet* 2:93–95.

Pickering, G. 1955. *High Blood Pressure*. New York: Grune and Stratton.

Pickering, G. 1968. *High Blood Pressure*. 2nd ed. New York: Grune and Stratton.

Pliskin, J. S., and Beck, C. H., Jr. 1976. A health index for patient selection: a value function approach—with application to chronic renal failure patients. *Management Science* 22:1009–1021.

Podell, R. N. 1975. *Physician's Guide to Compliance in Hypertension*. West Point, Pennsylvania: Merck.

Pomerleau, O.; Bass, F.; and Crown, V. 1975. Role of behavior modification in preventive medicine. *N. Engl. J. Med.* 292: 1277–1282.

Quetsch, R. M.; Achor, R. W. P.; Litin, E. M.; and Faucett, R. L. 1959. Depressive reactions in hypertensive patients: a comparison of those treated with Rauwolfia and those receiving no specific antihypertensive treatment. *Circulation* 19:366–375.

Raiffa, H. 1968. *Decision Analysis: Introductory Lectures on Choices under Uncertainty*. Reading, Massachusetts: Addison-Wesley.

Rehman, O. U.; Keith, T. A.; and Gall, E. A. 1973. Methyldopa-induced submassive hepatic necrosis. *J.T.M.A.* 224:1390–1392.

Robbins, S. L. 1967. *Pathology*. Philadelphia: Saunders.

Sackett, D. L. 1974. Screening for disease: cardiovascular diseases. *Lancet* 2:1189–1191.

Sackett, D. L.; Haynes, R. B.; Gibson, E. S.; Hackett, B.; Taylor, D. W.; Roberts, R. S.; and Johnson, A. L. 1975. Randomised clinical trial of strategies for improving medication compliance in primary hypertension. *Lancet* 1:1205–1207.

Sackett, D. L.; Spitzer, W. O.; Gent, M.; and Roberts, R. S. 1974. The Burlington randomized trial of the nurse practitioner: health outcomes of patients. *Ann. Intern. Med.* 80:137–142.

Schoenberger, J. A.; Stamler, J.; Shekelle, R. B.; and Shekelle, S. 1972. Current status of hypertension control in an industrial population. *J.A.M.A.* 222:559–562.

Schuster, S. R., and Gross, R. E. 1962. Surgery for coarctation of the aorta: a review of 500 cases. *J. Thorac. Cardiovasc. Surg.* 43:54–70.

Shaper, A. G. 1972. Cardiovascular disease in the tropics. Part 3: blood pressure and hypertension. *Br. Med. J.* 2:805–807.

Shapiro, A. P.; Benedek, T. G.; and Small, J. L. 1961. Effects of thiazides on carbohydrate metabolism in patients with hypertension. *N. Engl. J. Med.* 265:1028–1033.

Shepard, D., and Moseley, T. A. E. 1976. Mailed versus telephoned appointment reminders to reduce broken appointments in a hospital outpatient department. *Med. Care.* 14:268–273.

Shepard, D., and Zeckhauser, R. 1975. The assessment of programs to prolong life, recognizing their interaction with risk factors. Discussion paper no. 32 D. John F. Kennedy School of Government, Harvard University.

Silverberg, E., and Holleb, A. I. 1975. Major trends in cancer: twenty-five year survey. *Ca-A Cancer Journal for Clinicians* 25(1):2–7.

Sleisenger, M. H., and Fordtran, J. S. 1973. *Gastrointestinal Disease.* Philadelphia: Saunders.

Smith, W. M.; Thurm, R. H.; and Bromer, L. 1969. Comparative evaluation of Rauwolfia whole root and reserpine. *Clin. Pharmacol. Ther.* 10:338–343.

Social Security Administration. 1974a. (United States Department of Health, Education, and Welfare.) *Short-Stay Hospitals under Medicare, 1969: Use and Charges by 'Major Discharge Diagnosis, 1969.* Health Insurance Statistics HI-50. DHEW publication no. (SSA) 74–11702. Baltimore, Maryland.

Social Security Administration. 1974b. (United States Department of Health, Education, and Welfare.) *United States Population Projections for OASDHI Cost Estimates, Actuarial Study No. 72.* DHEW publication no. (SSA) 75–11518. Baltimore, Maryland.

Society of Actuaries, Committee on Mortality. 1959–1960. *Build and Blood Pressure Study.* Chicago.

Sokolow, M., and Perloff, D. 1960. Five-year survival of consecutive patients with malignant hypertension treated with antihypertensive agents. *Am. J. Cardiol.* 6:858–863.

Spitzer, W. O.; Sackett, D. L.; Sibley, J. C.; Roberts, R. S.; Gent, M.; Kergin, D. J.; Hackett, B. C.; and Olynich, A. 1974. The Burlington randomized trial of the nurse practitioner. *N. Engl. J. Med.* 290:251–256.

Stamler, R.; Stamler, J.; Civinelli, J.; Pritchard, D.; Gosch, F. C.; Ticho, S.; Restivo, B.; and Fine, D. 1975. Adherence and blood-pressure response to hypertension treatment. *Lancet* 2:1227–1230.

Starfield, B.; Sharp, E. S.; and Mellits, E. D. 1971. Effective care in the ambulatory setting: the nurse's contribution. *J. Pediatr.* 79:504–507.

Stokes, J. B., and Ward, G. W. 1974. The National High Blood Pressure Education Program. *Urban Health* 3:56+.

Stunkard, A. 1975. From explanation to action in psychosomatic medicine: the case of obesity. *Psychosom. Med.* 37:195–236.

Stunkard, A., and McLaren-Hume, M. 1959. The results of treatment of obesity. *Arch. Intern. Med.* 103:79–85.

Svarstad, B. 1974. The doctor-patient encounter: an observational study of communications and outcome. Ph.D. diss., Department of Sociology, University of Wisconsin.

Tagliacozzo, D. M. and Ima, K. 1970. Knowledge of illness as a predictor of patient behavior. *J. Chronic Dis.* 22:765–775.

Taylor, J. O. 1975. Personal communication.

Taylor, J. O. 1974. Personal communication.

Thorner, R. 1970. Strategy problems in disease prevention and their relationship to cost. In *Symposium on Early Disease Detection—What and How* (Elkhart, Indiana). Sponsored by Ames Co., Inc. Mt. Kisco, New York: Futura.

Time. 1975. 13 January, pp. 60–64.

Toghill, P. J.; Smith, P. G.; Benton, P.; Brown, R. C.; and Matthews, H. L. 1974. Methyldopa liver damage. *Br. Med. J.* 3:545–548.

Torrance, G. W.; Sackett, D. L.; and Thomas, W. H. 1973. Utility maximization model for program evaluation: a demonstration application. In *Health Status Indexes: Proceedings of a Conference Conducted by Health Services Research, Tucson, Arizona, 1972,* ed. R. L. Berg. Chicago: Hospital Research and Educational Trust.

Veterans Administration Cooperative Study Group on Antihypertensive Agents. 1972. Effects of treatment on morbidity in hypertension. Part 3. *Circulation* 45:991–1004.

Veterans Administration Cooperative Study Group on Antihypertensive Agents. 1970. Effects of treatment on morbidity in hypertension. Part 2. *J.A.M.A.* 213:1143–1152.

Veterans Administration Cooperative Study Group on Antihypertensive Agents. 1967. Effects of treatment on morbidity in hypertension. Part 1. *J.A.M.A.* 202:1028–1034.

Weisbrod, B. A. 1961. *Economics of Public Health.* Philadelphia: University of Pennsylvania Press.

Whitby, L. G. 1974. Screening for disease: definitions and criteria. *Lancet* 2:819–822.

Wilber, J. A., and Barrow, J. G. 1972. Hypertension—a community problem. *Am. J. Med.* 52:653–663.

Williamson, J. W. 1965. Assessing clinical judgment. *J. Med. Educ.* 40:180–187.

Worlledge, S. M.; Carstairs, K. C.; and Dacie, J. V. 1966. Autoimmune haemolytic anaemia associated with alpha-methyldopa therapy. *Lancet* 2:135–139.

Zinner, S. H.; Martin, L. F.; Sacks, F.; Rosner, B.; and Kass, E. H. 1974. A longitudinal study of blood pressure in childhood. *Am J. Epidemiol.* 100:437–442.

Index